CANCER STORIES
Creativity and Self-Repair

Psychoanalytic Inquiry Book Series

Volume 11

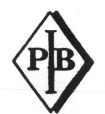

Psychoanalytic Inquiry
Book Series

CANCER STORIES
Creativity and
Self-Repair

Esther Dreifuss-Kattan

THE ANALYTIC PRESS

1990   Hillsdale, NJ   Hove and London

Published by The Analytic Press, Inc., Hillsdale, NJ.

Distributed solely by

Lawrence Erlbaum Associates, Inc., Publishers
365 Broadway
Hillsdale, New Jersey   07642

All literary excerpts, poems, and artwork reproduced herein are
reprinted with the generous permission of their copyright holders
and are appropriately credited in the Reference section at the end
of the volume.

Library of Congress Cataloging-in-Publication Data

Dreifuss-Kattan, Esther.
  Cancer stories : creativity and self-repair / Esther
  Dreifuss-Kattan.
  p.   cm. -- (Psychoanalytic Inquiry book series ; v. 11)
  Includes bibliographical references and index.
ISBN 0-88163-113-2
  1. Cancer--Psychological aspects. 2. Psychotherapy. 3.
  Psychoanalysis. 4. Creative writing- Therapeutic use.
  I. Title.   II. Series.
RC271.P79D74   1990
616.99'4'0019--dc20   90-46491
                                                   CIP

Printed in United States of America
10 9 8 7 6 5 4 3 2 1

*In memory of two men,
both highly creative,
both surprised by cancer:*

*My father, Max Dreifuss,
and my teacher, Fritz Meerwein.*

Renouncement. This is not what illness
    was
in childhood's days. A respite.
    Subterfuge
for growing. Things called and whispered
    promises.
Don't mix that old astonishment with
    this.

                                        —Rilke (1966, p. 354)

But it turns out that you can live a lifetime in a day; you can live
a lifetime in a moment; you can live a lifetime in a year—so that
to the extent they can prolong your life dying is not a lie. It's
something that's beautiful. I don't think people are afraid of
death. What they are afraid of is the incompleteness of their
life.

                                        —Rosenthal (1973, p. 45)

CONTENTS

ACKNOWLEDGMENTS

This work is itself an acknowledgment of the debt I owe to my late friend, teacher, and mentor, Professor Fritz Meerwein, M.D., teaching and training psychoanalyst at the Freud Institute in Zurich and founder and director of the Psychiatric Liaison Service at the Department for Internal Medicine at Zurich University Hospital. He guided me through the fields of psychooncology and psychoanalysis, and his creative questions, criticisms, support, and suggestions provided me with the stimulus to write this work.

I am also thankful to Professor George Martz, M.D., who headed the Department of Oncology at Zurich University Hospital and who supported art therapy as an integral part of the psychosocial liaison services as early as 1979. My thanks also to my teachers, Edith Kramer, A.T.R., H.L.M., a pioneer art therapist and artist, from New York University, and Penelope Williamson, Sc.D., and Marvin Surkin, Ph.D., both from The Union Institute in Cincinnati, Ohio, for their warm, consistent support throughout my studies and writing. I received valuable help from my friend Toby Moystesser, Ph.D., in editing as I struggled with English as a second language, and Olive Simone and Chris Price in typing my manuscript, and from my students Onn Ychilov, M.A., and Michal Falkan Navon, M.A., of Tel Aviv University, for their truly helpful research assistance. My gratitude to John Kerr of The Analytic Press for being a supportive, encouraging, and helpful guide in the preparation of this book.

Lots of thanks also to my husband, Shlomo, for his tolerant support and my two little girls, Sarit Yolanda and Gabriela Caroline, for their patience when Mummy was writing.

The warmest thanks to my patients who allowed me to be with them on their final journey.

PREFACE

Acknowledgment of the importance of psychosocial medicine has grown steadily over the last few years. The psychology of the cancer patient, in particular, not only has moved into the center of public attention, but also has become a serious subject of psychomedical research. The significance of such developmental psychodynamic concepts as defense and adaptation mechanisms; the role of unconscious fears, wishes, and fantasies; and the importance of the recognition and evaluation of feelings of depression and other psychosocial influences in the development of health and illness are all more and more recognized by traditional medicine and particularly in oncology.

The technical advances achieved in the treatment of cancer, which frequently result in cure or prolonged survival, are, however, often accompanied by a chronic disease process. Cancer treatments executed by highly specialized professionals, each having a share in the patient's care, heighten the fear and bewilderment of the patient, who is already forced to deal with the threat of the diagnosis and who faces numerous losses and discomforts. Today there is growing recognition of the emotional impact of cancer and its treatment on the quality of life of the patient and perhaps even on the outcome of the disease.

Moreover, cancer is seen by many as the typical representation of illness and dying, exemplified in the numerous autobiographical accounts written by cancer patients, many of which I have collected over the last five years and analyze in this volume.

In the first, psychooncological, part of this study, patients' perceptions of information sharing and the decision-making process, of the doctor-patient relationship and the various treatment methods, and of their own fears and pain in all phases of the illness are analyzed from the perspective of 32 published first-person accounts. Their interpretation is based on the classic work *Einfuehrung in die Psychooncologie (Introduction to Psychooncology)*, edited by the Swiss psychooncologist and psychoanalyst Fritz Meerwein, M.D. (1985a). This part of the book is addressed not only to the psychoanalyst, psychiatrist, and psychologist, but also to the oncologist, the primary care physician, other treatment team members, and the families who care for cancer patients.

The second part of my study investigates psychoanalytic concepts of mourning, loss, and creativity as they relate to the literature and art created by writers and artists who suffer from cancer. Writing and creating are interpreted in terms of psychological self-repair in the face of multiple losses and as reparation in view of one's own death, that is, as a means of unconsciously connecting with an intact inner good object. This analysis then serves as a theoretical framework informing various clinical issues in psychotherapeutic and art psychotherapeutic work with cancer patients and their families and is illustrated with case material and pictorial representations. I advance clinical considerations for the mobilization of the latent creativity of the cancer patient, paralleling that which develops spontaneously in the cancer author or artist, as a potent aid in the work of grieving and mourning.

Personal narratives, autobiographies, diaries, novels, poetic accounts, and art by authors, artists, and untrained patients who suffer cancer prove to be a rich source for identifying the major concerns of all cancer patients. The responses of creative people to a life-threatening disease offer great insight into our understanding of how human beings face loss and death and of the powerful, critical role creative work can play in this process. These cancer stories also highlight the importance of key therapeutic relationships for the patient doing the difficult work of mourning. The study concludes with a bibliography of 110 titles of books published by cancer authors in the last 20 years in English and in German.

All quotations from German and Swiss authors have been translated by the author.

—— 1 ——

Introduction

to

Psychooncology

*"In literature . . . there alone, the condition can be
fulfilled which makes it possible for us to reconcile
ourselves with death. . . ."*

(Freud, 1915, p. 291)

Every historical period has an illness that especially frightens it. In Biblical
times, it was leprosy that provoked the deepest disgust and fear. In the
Middle Ages and during the Renaissance, the "black death" was the
unstoppable, devastating demon. In Florence, for example, 60,000 inhab-
itants died of plague in one year, a calamity that inspired Giovanni
Boccaccio to write *The Decameron*. In the 19th century, the "white death,"
tuberculosis, was associated with the greatest suffering; against it no
weapon was strong enough. In *The Magic Mountain*, Thomas Mann wrote
of the tuberculosis patient, consumed by illness. He described the illness's
visible symptoms and the patient's particular psychic makeup. Before the
discovery that TB is a bacterial infection, the TB patient was always a
terminal patient.

Today cancer is the illness that evokes the most intense fears. The
word cancer can be traced to Hippocrates, who linked the long, distant
veins radiating from lumps in the breast to crabs. Cancers, like crabs, creep
in unpredictable, sideways motions, hidden from view, like primitive
animals of the night. Like the crab protected by its shell, cancer is
aggressive yet unattackable; it inflicts pain and holds tenaciously to what
it seizes. Devouring and destroying, it has the death of its victim as its goal.

In 1798 the German writer Novalis described cancerous tumors as "full-fledged parasites, they grow, are engendered, engender, have structure, secrete and eat" (cited in Sontag, 1979, p. 13). Freud called his oral cavity cancer his "monster" (Schur, 1972). "The cancer patient shrivels," wrote Alice James (1964, p. 225) in her journal, a year before she died of breast cancer, which she called "this unholy granite substance in my breast" (p. 225).

No other disease attracts to itself such a wealth of personal symbols and metaphorical equivalences. One has but to hear the diagnosis "cancer" to begin imagining a slow process of bodily destruction and inevitable death. The idea that cancer is a physical condition, one that frequently can be arrested or even cured, is psychologically beyond reach. Instead, a picture of a slow, wasting death emerges and is promptly interpreted in terms of one's life to date. A heart attack is just a heart attack, but cancer is a punishment for a life poorly lived or for suppressed hostility, or else it is the culmination of one's hopelessness. These and other personal interpretations invariably color one's perception of the illness. They are not the result of an inadvertent suggestion by a doctor or nurse. Each patient makes the interpretation instantly. So, too, does the patient's family, though often the family's metaphor is significantly different from the patient's.

It is important for the doctor and the patient to elicit these metaphors and to understand that, in each case, the interpretation of the cancer has been filtered through the patient's perceptions, personality, and total life experience. The oncologist's first questions to the patient should always be, What gave you the illness? What fantasies do you have about why you have it? To hear the answer to these questions is to become immediately acquainted with the person standing in front of you.

As the cancer patient and writer Maxi Wander (1980) described in her diary, "To think of cancer is like being locked up in a room with a murderer. You never know when, where, how and if he will attack you" (p. 15).

Psychooncology tries to deal therapeutically with the psychological realities behind these metaphors and with the defenses that the patient and doctor employ against these overpowering images. It examines the psychological responses to the various cancer therapies and their consequences for the patient, the family, and the treatment team. It also deals with the threat of death and other fears that the patient experiences from the onset and throughout all the stages of his illness.

Thomas Percival wrote in his *Medicinal Ethics*, published in 1803: "The feelings and emotions of patients under critical circumstances, require to be known and to be attended to, no less than the symptoms of their diseases" (cited in Meerwein, 1980, p. 13). In the last several years, psychooncology has received increasing public attention and gained its place in scientific, medical, and psychological research. The following reasons explain these developments:

—Cancer constitutes the second most prevalent cause of human death.

—Advances in surgical, radiotherapeutic, and chemotherapeutic treatment methods have extended the life of cancer patients and in many cases increased the chances of cure. At the same time, however, these advantages have greatly influenced the quality of survivors' lives and they often become chronic patients.

—Patients have the right, and need, to be an active partner in their own illness. They wish to be involved in the decision-making process leading to the selection of various medical procedures.

—Today's patients expect their treatment plan to include a fight against fear. They know that only a more or less fear-free personality is sufficiently strong to fight and win the war against cancer.

—Cancer is usually a slow process, in which one can observe psychic development over a long period of time.

The metaphor cancer, however, contains a strange paradox. Cancer, or *carcinoma* in Latin, means tumor; in Greek, *neoplasma*, which means "forming of the new." The threat of destruction that this "new" tissue represents invariably evokes dread, but in many patients it also rouses dormant energies as both physical and psychological resources are tapped to fight the illness. Often, in an effort to restore health and regain one's psychic balance, new creative forces are found. Thus a unique dialectic emerges between illness and health, between despair and new hope. The fact of having cancer, as we shall see in the many autobiographical and artistic accounts that follow, can evoke in many patients a strong wish for self-expression. "If my slow dying, which cannot be doubted any longer, is preordained, then I have only one last wish: that I can make out of this dying, a beautiful, great exciting story," wrote the Swiss cancer patient and author W.M. Diggelmann (1979) in his last book, *Shadows* (p. 28).

I use the term "cancer stories" to designate published writings by cancer patients that deal with any of the various aspects of their illnesses. These include autobiographies, diaries, personal narratives, novels, and poetry, as well as several scientific studies written by psychologists, psychoanalysts, physicians, and philosophers whose cancer motivated them to write scientific inquires on the impact of cancer and its life threat.

Most, but not all, of the cancer authors were writers before their illness. Using diaries or dictaphones, they started to document their cancer. They were driven by a range of motives created by the illness.

Some, like Diggelmann (1979), started writing in order to keep control of their lives despite the ravages of their illness:

> It was my only way, the only weapon I had to fight the illness. So I arranged for this dictaphone six weeks ago. Because I told myself, whatever happens to you, you're not going to give up. You're going to change it. You're going to make something out of it. You're going to have to use your imagination. It's no use curling up and playing dead [p. 102].

Others, such as the young physician Fitz Mullan (1987), were motivated by the desire to leave something of themselves behind:

> When at the age of thirty-two I was diagnosed as having cancer, my parents gave me a hand held tape recorder and suggested I use what energy I could muster to keep notes on my ordeal. Writing was my art, something I had done a great deal of and enjoyed. Keep a diary, they suggested. Maybe it will make a book someday. I think we all doubted that. More likely my jottings would make a memento, some final tracks in the sand if I went on to die as was the strong possibility. That rationale was not offensive to me. In fact it made sense and I set about a daily dictation describing hospital life and my adjustment to it as a cancer patient [p. 45].

The cancer book or work of art provides the cancer patient with a projection screen for all the fears provoked by the disease. Betty Rollin, the television journalist, (1976) writes:

> I was still going to the office during my crazy time, and going out at night, too. I don't think my craziness showed much. That was partly because I was writing more, now, and putting my craziness down on paper. That made it more possible to be sane the rest of the time. Sometimes I reminded myself of one of those people who goes berserk and kills fourteen people from a rooftop and afterwards the neighbors say, "But he was such a quiet boy. So polite." Then they find this loony diary [p. 156].

The creative work of the cancer patient often becomes the container for all the shifting emotions, especially fear and grief, that are experienced in the course of the illness and treatment, as Audre Lorde (1980), the American poet, wrote:

October 10, 1987

I want to write about the pain. The pain of waking up in the recovery room which is worsened by that immediate sense of loss. Of going in and out of pain and shots. Of the correct position for my arm to drain. The euphoria of the 2nd day, and how it's been downhill from there.

I want to write of the pain I am feeling right now, of the lukewarm tears that will not stop coming into my eyes—for what? For my lost breast? For the lost me? And which me was that again anyway? For the death I don't know how to postpone? Or how to meet elegantly? [p.24].

The work of art or literature enables the cancer patient to objectify and externalize, and hence to communicate, the realities of the illness, from the emotions it involves through the details of the treatments, realities that are difficult to communicate face to face: "It only remained for me to give it voice, to share it for use, that the pain not be wasted," Lorde (1980, p. 16) put it succinctly. Like all literature and art, the production of the cancer patient fulfills the need for self-expression and enhances communication; the fact of cancer both gives urgency to the need for expression and places obstacles in the way of more direct communication.

Cancer patients often feel that they want to write about pain, loss, and fear till "he owns the experience," as Nancy Fried, a New York sculptor (cited in Langer, 1989, p. 133), put it after her mastectomy. Or, as Eva Hesse, the American artist who died at the age of 34 of a malignant brain tumor, said, "If something is meaningful, maybe it's more meaningful said ten times" (cited in Langer, 1989, p. 133).

By writing, the patient battles against the feeling that the cancer is totally senseless and deprives life of meaning. Most of the cancer authors discussed in this book were in midlife and describe how cancer intruded into their lives too early and threatened to destroy them. Writing is the cancer author's answer to the meaninglessness inherent in death. Paradoxically, the creative assertion of meaning in the face of death is made possible by one's essential inability to grasp fully and to come to terms with one's own death. Freud pointed out this inability in 1915 when he wrote, "It is indeed impossible to imagine our own death and whenever we attempt to do so we can perceive that we are in fact still present as spectators . . . that in the unconscious every one of us is convinced of his own immortality" (p. 289). Cancer authors frequently express the impossibility of imagining their own nonexistence. For example, Peter Noll (1984), a Professor of Law at Zurich University in his 50s, writes,

"Sometimes a funny thought follows me, that I will continue living for another five to ten years, as a medical miracle. . . . We are forced to live as if we were immortal" (p.34). Similarly, Stewart Alsop (1973), a well-known journalist also in his 50s, writes,

> When I began to write this book, I accepted John's [the doctor] odds, 20–1 against more than two years of life. Suppose I last much longer? I can imagine rude whispered comments: "Isn't that old creep the man who wrote about how he was dying of cancer?" Curious, the prospect of being embarrassed to be still alive [p. 270].

By writing, the cancer patient retains the role of "spectator" of his own death. He is not merely the principal actor in the drama of his dying; he is also the primary audience. In the act of writing down his experiences, the author achieves a distance from the brutalities of the illness. As the cancer author Sikes (1984) states, the goal is "to see myself from the outside, as a character in my own life" (p. 308). By adopting the spectator's position, the cancer author is finally able to confront the grim truth of his own and all human mortality. As Noll (1984) writes:

> I wanted to describe death and dying as an unavoidable event each of us has to go through and overcome, to show my own situation as our common lot, but at the same time as an example. I wanted to show the reader that to confront death, dying and fantasies of afterlife while still alive makes a lot of sense [p. 227].

Among its many other functions, then, the cancer book serves its author as a means of coping with, and perhaps overcoming, the universal terror of dying. Lorde (1980) expressed this function quite explicitly: "And I began to recognize a source of power within myself that comes from the knowledge that while it is most desirable not to be afraid, learning to put fear into perspective gave me great strength" (p. 20).

The cancer authors discussed in this book all offer personal interpretations, not factual records, of what happened during their illness. The remembered material is arranged in a personal sequence and is subject to the fictionalizing processes of selection and omission. This autobiographical act not only confers a new formal quality upon the experience, which the original illness never had, but also enables the author to reevaluate his illness and to give it meaning. By selectively writing down and shaping such an overwhelming experience, the patient is able to integrate it and give it coherence. Cancer literature is generally characterized by a dialectic play of distance and intimacy that makes this kind of writing distinctive as a mode of self-knowledge.

The feeling of distance derives from the cancer narrator's stance as a reflective observer, while the sense of intimacy derives from the narrator's being the chief protagonist of the threatening drama he discloses. Writing about the fear and the pain of loss is itself a process of accepting and overcoming these emotions. The cancer author confronts his adversity and his new self; this confrontation is an affirmation of life. To achieve that affirmation, the patient must always fight against his self-protective defenses. The struggle is described in many of the cancer books I have read. The following admission by Lorde (1980) is only one of many statements to this effect:

> This reluctance is a reluctance to deal with myself, with my own experiences and the feelings buried in them and the conclusions to be drawn from them. It is also, of course, a reluctance to living or reliving, giving life or new life to that pain [p. 25].

Cancer forces a patient to modify his entire life plan. We often find in cancer books an account of the life of the author up to the diagnosis (that is, his previous life plan), and then its reexamination. The patient tries to reformulate a new life plan in accordance with his new situation, which is continuously changing according to the course and limitations imposed by his chronic or terminal illness. For example, a drawn-out disease course often enforces a new life-style or a new constellation of associates, and some cancer books describe the author's search for a new community. To a certain extent, the loss of part of the old life plan also means a loss of identity. The cancer stories thus are often accounts of finding a new identity, of becoming a new person.

As we shall see in the following 31 personal accounts of cancer authors, the cancer literature contains moving depictions of illness, dying, and creativity and demonstrates how we are all interconnected, the sick and the healthy, and how losses bind and embrace us all.

PART I

Psychooncological Analysis of the Cancer Literature

2

THE EARLY PHASE

OF

CANCER

The chronic nature of cancer causes the patient and his family, as well as his doctors and the health care team, great emotional tension. Some of this tension may be mitigated by a step-by-step approach. In the following pages, I discuss the phases and treatment methods of cancer insofar as they relate to the doctor-patient relationship. My hope is that an understanding of the course of cancer, as it affects the patient's psychology and is described by the cancer patient author, will help the physician and other members of the treatment team to avoid an overidentification with the patient that would stand in the way of an objective, empathic, clinical stance. In this chapter, I present a description of the correlation of physical and psychological developments during the prediagnostic and diagnostic phases early in the course of the illness.

PREDIAGNOSTIC PHASE

The prediagnostic phase begins when the patient consults the doctor for a routine check-up or presents certain symptoms that, subjectively or objectively, arouse a suspicion of cancer. In a survey of 76 female patients with a suspicious breast condition, 73% made a correct evaluation of their illness before the actual diagnosis (Schwartz, 1984). Even if a "healthy" person comes to the doctor for a routine physical examination, it is important to ask, what prompted you to ask for this checkup just now? Behind the request, the patient often hides a secret, denied fear of cancer that needs to be uncovered and dealt with.

DELAY IN SEEKING DIAGNOSIS

Delays occur when patients, who sense from some inner perception that they may have cancer, manage to put off having the illness diagnosed by a physician. Patients usually find reasons for their procrastination. Some rush to consult the doctor in order to relieve anxiety, but others will wait and wait. Most patients, however, delay no more than about eight weeks after the initial symptoms appear, regardless of the site (Hackett, Cassem, and Raker, 1973) For certain types of cancer, a delay in diagnosis of three or more months increases the chances of death from cancer by 10 to 20%.

The reasons for postponing an examination are as complicated as human nature itself, as Weisman (1979) has pointed out. The following are some of them: (1) the incorrect assumption that cancer is always a terminal illness; (2) past experiences with family or friends who had cancer; (3) painless symptoms, disregarded under the popular assumption that cancer is always painful; (4) latent suicidal tendencies in older, depressed patients who have poor insurance coverage and fear high medical costs; (5) fear of a physical examination in shy and timid people; (6) fear of hospitals and operations; and (7) a poor doctor–patient relationship. Old people, poorly educated people, and people of lower socioeconomic status tend to delay more than others.

Physicians sometimes contribute to delaying the cancer diagnosis, though precisely how frequently is not known. The motive for professional delay is often the physician's repressed overidentification with a cancer patient. Such repression may lead the physician to conspire with the young patient's own wish for delay. Similarly, it may augment the physician's fear of injuring (through surgical intervention) a highly libidinal organ, a danger that can mobilize unconscious "castration fears," which the physician needs to repress. Whatever the motive, however, the patient is always the victim when diagnosis is delayed.

The following passages by Rollin (1976) describe a blatant conspiracy to delay the cancer diagnosis:

> I had a lump for a year. At least a year. It was a hard little thing-about the size of a yellow grape—and it resided, imperceptible except to the touch, on the far left side of my left breast, due west of the nipple. I knew it was there, my (ex-)husband knew it was there, my (ex-)internist knew it was there, and my (ex-)mammographer knew it was there. Of the four, only one of us was worried about it. That was Arthur Herzog [the husband], who had found it on a spring evening in 1974 during a routine sexual feel.

"What's that?" he said. "I don't know," I said. "It's a lump," he said. "Mmmmm," I said, wanting to sleep. "Will you get it looked at?" he said. "Sure," I said, and went to sleep. I got it looked at. "It's nothing to worry about," said my internist on Central Park West, whom I'll call Dr. Smith. "Feels like a cyst. A lot of women have them. But we'll send you for some mammograms."

I went for some mammograms. "This doesn't worry me a bit," said my mammographer on East Ninetieth Street, whom I'll call Dr. Ellby. He held up his pictures of my lump to the light. "Come back in a year and we'll have another look. . . ."

Whew. Not that I had been worried, either. Well, maybe just a little. Anyway, I was glad to be out of there . . . [pp. 3–4]

Rollin goes on to say:

For almost a year, that was that. Although I did not worry about the lump, I could not entirely forget about it, either. It was, after all, there. Once in a while I'd feel it—sort of push it in with my index finger. It was an absentminded gesture, the way one feels a mole or a callus. Still there? Oh, well, isn't it nice that it doesn't mean anything [p. 7].

She continues:

Besides, piped up my unconscious, you're a reporter. You're immune. You're doing a story about women with a possible affliction, you're not one of them. You're—the word is "covering" them—on the outside. You're a journalist. You've got credentials, press passes to get into places, or out. You can get assistance when you need it, or protection, if you need that. You're special. You're safe. You note screams in your spiral notebook, but they never come from your own throat [p. 8].

Rollin tells us:

I went back to Dr. Ellby before the year was up. My first visit had been in June, 1974. Now it was late March, 1975. "That's my lump," I said when he got to it. He looked at me. "I had it a year ago. You said it was nothing and that I should come back in a year." I was annoyed at having to explain.

He nodded and drew a black circle around the lump with a pen. "That'll wash off," he said and walked out [pp. 14–15].

After Dr. Ellby performed the mammography, he asked the patient to call her physician to receive the results.

> I flipped the Rolodex to Dr. Smith's number, stared at it for about ten seconds, and decided to let myself be a pest.
>
> "I'm sorry to bother you," I said when he came to the phone, "But I was at Ellby's yesterday, and he said if anything were wrong, he'd call you, so I guess he hasn't, but I just thought I'd check because I'm probably going out of town. . . ."
>
> He did not speak immediately, and when he spoke he pronounced each word as if he had had a rehearsal. The words I remember were ". . . nothing to worry about, but it really should come out."
>
> I didn't speak right away, either. "When?"
>
> "I'll give you the number of a surgeon. Dr. Singermann—he's first-rate. Make an appointment with him and he'll do the rest."
>
> "Does it have to be right away?" I was vaguely alarmed, but mostly it sounded like another annoyance, more time wasted—as if the Dr. Ellby business weren't enough. Still, I wasn't expecting this. "I'm going to California for a week. Is it—should I try to get back sooner—I mean, how serious is it?"
>
> "The end of the week would be just fine, Betty," said Dr. Smith, not really answering my question. "Look," he added, when he realized I was hanging on for more, "Most of these things are benign. It just seems like a good idea to have it out. OK?" [pp. 18–19].

The doctor's tendency to identify with a patient in the same age group as he is quite prevalent, and the result is always to the disadvantage of the patient. Doctors also tend to delay as a way of disguising their own concerns. Robbins, McDonald, and Pack (1983) studied 229 doctors who had cancer and saw that the doctors had the same tendency to procrastinate after they recognized the first symptoms as did the average nonmedical population. Physicians often go to the most unsuitable colleague for an examination.

Such a physician was Sigmund Freud. In 1923, when he was 66 years old, Freud showed a lesion in his mouth to his friend and doctor, Dr. Felix Deutsch. Deutsch immediately recognized what he saw as an advanced cancer but decided to tell Freud that the lesion was a leukoplatia. Deutsch suggested that it be operated on by Hajek, a professor of laryngology whom observers had judged "a surgeon of surprising mediocrity" (Romm, 1983, p. 709). Freud delayed his visit to the surgeon for two months. Finally, Hajek performed an incomplete excision of Freud's tumor, followed by highly inadequate postoperative care. Because of an unforeseen blood loss, Hajek was forced to admit Freud to the hospital, but a proper bed was unavailable and Freud was put in a small, auxiliary room with an imbecile, deaf-mute dwarf. Shortly afterward, when his daughter and his wife, who learned about the operation only after the patient had to be hospitalized, left for lunch, Freud suffered a severe hemorrhage. According to his biographer, Ernest Jones (1957),

> to get help, he rang the bell, which was out of order: he himself could neither speak nor call out. The friendly dwarf, however, rushed for help and after a while the bleeding was stopped: perhaps the dwarf's good offices saved Freud's life. He was weak due to loss of blood, was half-drugged by the medicines, and was in great pain. During the night, she [his daughter Anna] and the nurse became alarmed at his condition and sent for the house surgeon who, however, refused to get out of bed [pp. 90–91].

Hajek appeared the following morning only to demonstrate Freud's case to a group of students and to dismiss him from the hospital. Hajek left no record of the operation, made no arrangements for further surgery, and did not inform his patient of the persistence of residual cancer. As Romm, a plastic surgeon, describes, Hajek's management of the case must, by available evidence, be judged as negligently deficient. Even though his cancer had only just begun (it lasted 16 years), Freud was deceived by his friends and his doctor, and he in turn deceived his family, delayed his treatment, and accepted deplorable medical and nursing care. Only after the growth in his mouth recurred and further surgery became necessary did Freud find a good surgeon and obtain proper medical care. According to Golub (1981), "although Freud would have been the first to acknowledge denial of death . . . as an adaptive defense, it would seem that it does not facilitate high quality medical treatment" (p. 81).

A contemporary physician, Alan Stoudemire (1983), describes his procrastination in checking out the persistent pain in his leg:

> The pain gradually continued. I kept promising that "I'd get somebody to take a look at it." I had, however, already self-diagnosed the pain, which occurred at the anterior aspect of my right tibia, as tendonitis. I presented the case in this way to one of my residents, who agreed with my diagnosis and advised me to take aspirin. I did take aspirin, which relieved the pain temporarily; however, I eventually noted that a tender mass was developing over the painful area. I then got a

"curbside" consultation from another resident, who after mulling it over for a while, thought I might have "a little osteomalacia" and said, "You might want to get it x-rayed sometime."

Five months after the onset of the pain, the entire knee became swollen and extremely painful. I was unable to walk on it. Again, I asked a medical resident to check it. He ordered an x-ray. The x-ray film looked as if "something" had literally devoured my anterior tibia. Still, the thought of cancer was rigidly repressed; I did not even think of the possibility. I referred myself to the staff clinic at the city teaching hospital, where the resident made a diagnosis of osteoid osteoma, a benign lesion. It was not benign. When the attending surgeon finally saw the x-ray, he knew it was cancer [p. 380].

Like Freud, Stoudemire at first chose unfit doctors to examine him; and like Freud's doctors, they, too, denied the seriousness of his problem in an overidentification with their sick colleague.

3

Psychological Reactions to the Diagnosis of Cancer

For all their reluctance to know about their cancer in the pre-diagnostic phase, many cancer patients sense their illness. Francoise Prevost (1976), a famous French actress, consciously denied the possibility that the tumor in her breast might indeed be cancerous, but her unconscious perceived and communicated this knowledge through a dream:

> My wonderful optimism, as foolish as it was, helped me get through a few days without churning too many problems around in my head. I convinced myself that I had a cyst and pushed the thought that I had cancer far out of my mind. The border, however, that separates the conscious from the unconscious is like a sheet of glass armor, transparent but impossible to pass through. Our dreams sometimes push through and transmit in some strange way the coded messages of our ego. It was indeed a dream that threw me back into doubts and fears.
>
> I was on a crowded street. A woman without a breast was walking next to me. She had forgotten to get dressed and was wearing only a skirt and shoes. Everyone was looking at her. I was embarrassed for her and, terrified, I tried to hide her. I also tried to talk to her, to tell her that she should put something on, that she should go into some building, that she should just disappear. But I couldn't get a sound out of my mouth. Even though I tried desperately to talk, she heard nothing and

merely smiled at me. We went into a fur shop. Coats were lying around all over, and she tried on every one of them while the salesman and customers looked on petrified.

Wearing a fox shawl she turned about and moved like a model and showed everybody her naked chest and her scars. She seemed very happy and kept smiling [p. 60].

Being an actress, Prevost had to rehearse her breast amputation in her dream before she was psychologically prepared to be operated on. The dream helped her to confront reality.

Cancer sufferers show a range of responses as they become aware of their possible disease. Dora Hauri (1982), a 28-year-old Swiss woman, after initial uncertainty and some denial, took responsibility for having her symptoms checked out, as she describes in her diary:

November 16th, 1978
    Knot in the breast.
    No period.
    Tiredness.
    What was it? The smoking? The drinking? The addiction to movement? My rearing up in protest? A spurt of flame? [p. 9].

December 10th, 1978
    Yesterday I visited the doctor, he was damned honest with me; it could be something serious, maybe not, but the possibility is there. I have to go to the hospital on Tuesday; I cried a lot [p. 11].

Hauri reacts with sadness. She starts to ask questions and to search for answers.

Noll (1984) exhibited a very different reaction when he heard the diagnosis of progressed cancer of the bladder. He became depressed.

In the meantime I discovered that I am more and more in love with sleep . . . [p. 11]. I think about what went through my head when the urologist told me my diagnosis. . . . My main thought was: It is not worth it. It was for sure no shock. Also not later, more the feeling: bad luck, no rebellion, no despair. But the tumor absorbs not only my body but also my thoughts. It's always following me, sometimes unconsciously [p. 12].

These lines illustrate Noll's struggle with a reactive depression.

Alsop (1973) felt lonely and overwhelmed when he received his diagnosis of acute leukemia.

> In fact, I more than resented being left alone—I feared it. On the second page of my notebook, after the scribble "leukemia," there is a longer scribble: "Tish [wife] left briefly this afternoon and suddenly I was alone with an awful loneliness." Those words tell something about what it is like to have a killing cancer, especially at first [p. 53].

HOW TO TELL

The most frequent question asked about a newly diagnosed cancer is whether or not to tell the patient the truth. Truth is not easy to deal with, and it is often either diluted or relegated to someone else to tell. Some families may demand silence, deception, or conspiracy from the doctor. Findings by Weisman (1972), however, show that only 10% of newly diagnosed cancer patients do not want to know the facts of their illness. The rest want all the "truth."

After all the medical tests have been completed, the patient needs sufficient information from the physician to participate in the decision of treatment. An informed patient is a better patient. Truth contributes to better coping because doctors and patients then share a common reality. Cancer patients need to be familiar with the specific aspects of their illness and the proposed treatment plan. The presumption that "doctor knows best" and that the best patients ask no questions is outmoded. When a family insists on secrecy, it is often because of their own anguish; their demand for deception reflects poor family relationships. Suicide is extremely infrequent among cancer patients and seldom follows learning the diagnosis. Secrecy only bars effective communication and puts off coping. Distress is determined largely by how patients are told about cancer, not by what they are told. And most patients suspect the diagnosis anyway (Weisman, 1979).

The doctor needs a great deal of flexibility to be able to relate to each patient's particular situation and personality when relaying the diagnosis. He needs to be a sensitive listener. He must listen to what the patient already knows and understand the patient's fears and resistance. He should be sensitive to the patient's nonverbal communication. And he should also understand the coping strategies available for dealing with life-threatening illnesses. Finally, the doctor should also understand and accept his own fears of illness and dying. This awareness is vital to open discussion with the newly diagnosed cancer patient. When the doctor explains the diagnosis to patients and suggests a treatment plan, he needs, at the same time, to assure them that he will offer them support on the long road ahead.

Many doctors are ill at ease and, hence, unempathic in relating the diagnosis of cancer. The resulting coldness and discomfort can add to the horror and shock for the patient who is learning about his condition for the first time. The following account by Rollin (1976), who fainted after her doctor presented the tentative diagnosis, shows how vital a more humane approach is:

> I was on my back and Singermann [the surgeon] was palpating my left breast. "Put your arm back." More palpation. Then the other breast. The examination was more thorough than any I had had before, either by Smith or Ellby. "Sit up, please." More of the same. He moved my arm this way and that, then pushed his fingers into my armpit, as if he were going to pick me up. Then "I'm going to squeeze your nipple now," he said, and did. I knew that if you have breast cancer, the nipple sometimes ejects a fluid. Mine didn't. It didn't even hurt. "You can get dressed now," said Singermann, without a trace of anything dour in his voice. Clearly, I had done as well on the physical as I had on the oral exam.
>
> I flounced back into the chair in his office. Arthur was still in his chair, chain-smoking.
>
> I don't remember exactly how Singermann put it, because, as soon as I got the gist of what he was saying, my head seemed to fill with air and my eyes got hot. ". . . definitely something there . . . a mass . . . good chance of malignancy . . . different kinds of mastectomy, as you probably know. Some women say they want a separate procedure . . . studies show . . . in my own experience . . . but, of course, it's up to you."
>
> He stopped. I realized I was supposed to talk now. It sounded as if I was expected to say whether I wanted just to have my breast cut off, or whether I wanted my breast cut off and some other things too.
>
> Slowly, I turned in my chair and looked at Arthur. Our eyes locked. He told me later he was unable to get the look on my face out of his mind. Not wanting to be rude, I turned back to Singermann. I heard myself speak. "Are you saying that you think I have cancer?" (That word had not been used. I soon learned that cancer is a word doctors almost never use.) "I mean, I know you can't know for sure, but what are the odds— what percentage—what is the likelihood . . .?"

Dr. Singermann smiled and leaned on his desk. "Everyone wants numbers. It's very hard to say, maybe seventy-thirty, sixty-forty, I don't know."

I heard myself speak again. "Are you saying, do you mean it's sixty or seventy percent *likely*, you mean it's *likely*?" It was making him uncomfortable. "Look, percentages are just percentages. People want numbers, you give them numbers, but . . . unreliable . . . you don't really know until . . . but . . ." Then he stood up. Then Arthur stood up. Then I stood up. Then I fell down . . . [pp. 34-35].

Singermann had left the room after I fell. I heard his voice now from one of the other rooms outside. "You never know about these things. Her doctor said she could take it . . . Everybody wants you to be honest . . . and look what happens." I put my hands down, away from my face. ". . . very upset . . .," I heard Arthur say. "Sixty percent is just a number." That was Singermann [p. 36].

Christine Lenker (1984), a high-school teacher in her late 20s, similarly described her doctor's discomfort in communicating the diagnosis.

When the examination finally took place, I heard my doctor's voice as if through a fog: "We have to remove this." At that moment I knew I was a cancer patient. I started shaking and waited for an explanation, an elaboration, a statement that it wasn't so bad. But my doctor remained silent. That's why I asked after a while, "Is it malignant?" "Yes—99%." "Is it big?" "Yes, pretty big." Silence. "Today is Friday, I will try to find you a hospital bed by Monday, if not by Wednesday." Silence. "I'll call and let you know." Silence. Here it was, my first confrontation with my doctor who has learned to tell the truth, but not to acknowledge its threat. I was not angry because I realized how uncomfortable he felt and how much he seemed to suffer in this situation; who likes to tell a young woman that she has breast cancer?   [p. 15].

Like so many physicians, who may otherwise be highly competent in the technical matters of cancer treatment, Rollin's and Lenker's doctors missed the opportunity to establish a trusting relationship with their patients. The first interview should serve not only as a forum for presenting the bare facts of the diagnosis, but as the basis for initiating an ongoing doctor-patient relationship. An empathic approach not only helps the patient to deal with the diagnosis, but influences the relationship the patient can establish to the illness, the treatment, and the doctor.

REACTIONS TO DIAGNOSIS

The most common initial reactions to the diagnosis of cancer are disbelief and shock. The thought that it cannot be cancer may persist for days. The entire future is in question. Many patients are overwhelmed when they hear the diagnosis. Initially they have little means of adapting to their new reality. They are overcome by intense feelings, as we saw in the examples of Rollin and Lenker. Cancer, in contrast to most other diseases, is linked to death, and a diagnosis of cancer gives rise to strong fears and uncanny fantasies. The diagnosis of cancer is associated with a slow, painful dying that cannot be forestalled by treatment. Cancer is imagined as something bad growing inside oneself and devouring one from the inside. No other illness provokes such metaphorical thinking. The feelings of having something bad inside oneself and of already belonging to death are characteristic fantasies of cancer patients (see Hackett et al., 1973; Vollmoeller, 1982).

The Swiss writer Diggelmann (1979), who suffered from a brain tumor with metastases in the lungs, describes the diagnostic period on many different levels:

> The tests are completed quickly and the picture of my disease becomes clearer from hour to hour. The medical team works intensively on the diagnosis as if on a puzzle. Each doctor contributes his suggestions about what to do and what remains to be checked out. What bothers me is the fact, or the realization, that strangely enough nothing bothers me any longer. There is something in this room that makes me seem nonexistent. I can't see myself. I don't feel anything any more. I don't feel like talking about it any longer. I am not interested in my case any longer [p. 18].

Diggelmann withdraws emotionally as the threat that his illness will be diagnosed as terminal comes closer. But he does not deny the possible diagnosis. Even before the doctors verify it, his fantasies show how intensely involved he already is with death:

> At that time [childhood] I touched you as life with my wings and you rose to the heavens. Now my wings of death touch you. Are you ready to provide me with shelter, as when I came to you then? My gift today is a gift of death for the living. Give to the living your portion of death, in this way you give yourself a gift of life. Don't bother to understand it, just give me shelter in your room. Take me in, I am death and I am life. If

you don't take me, death, in, don't expect me to appeal to you again as life. . . . I don't beg as death for your life. I give you your life as a gift by coming to you as death. Don't push me away, don't defend yourself. . . . You will eventually realize that it is not death who knocks on your window, but transformed life [p. 21].

Confronted with the actual diagnosis, Diggelmann writes the following:

For days I have been sitting next to the window in the small gray room. The doctors, who mean well, tell me day after day how strong the bad death flower grows in my head, grows roots, how it feels comfortable in the safety of the wall of my skull. It is blooming beautifully, the doctors tell me, and it is very connected to me as if it loved me. At night, I sit in front of the black window and hear in the quiet of my long road to death the begging voice of a new flower . . . [p. 22].

Diggelmann's beautiful words do not diminish the tremendous fear he feels after learning of his brain tumor.

The anguish provoked by the cancer diagnosis can be seen in Alsop's (1973) account. Alsop's agony was exacerbated by the long time it took to reach a certain diagnosis, but his reaction is not otherwise atypical:

I wrote my letter as a takeoff on Winston's famous speech of defiance. "We will fight amongst the platelets," I wrote, "We will fight in the bone marrow. We will fight in the peripheral blood. We will never surrender."

Having written this, I began, for the first time in about fifty years, to cry. I was utterly astonished, and also dismayed. I was brought up to believe that for a man to weep in public is the ultimate indignity, a proof of unmanliness. Only my elderly roommate was in the room, and he hadn't noticed. I ducked into our tiny shared bathroom, and closed the door, and sat down on the toilet, and turned on the bath water, so that nobody could hear me, and cried my heart out. Then I dried my eyes on the toilet paper and felt a good deal better [p. 68].

With crying, Alsop could relieve some of the incredible tension that had built up in the diagnostic period.

In Mullan's (1985) book *Vital Signs: A Doctor's Struggle with Cancer*, we see the desperation that overcomes the physician as he admits to himself that the x-ray film he made of the chest cancer while working in the hospital was in fact his own:

> I had taken only a single view of my chest, assuming I would find nothing. I stuffed the plastic rectangle under the lip of the viewing box and peered into my own chest. My first glance told me that something was very wrong. To the right of the heart and confluent with its border was a fluffy white density that extended into all the lobes of the right lung. It was the size of a grapefruit, but on the X-ray looked like a hazy cauliflower.
>
> The physician in me responded first and I instinctively looked at the grim information on the viewing box as a clinician. This was an unusual finding, a fascinating X-ray, I said to myself. Here are a number of possibilities that will have to be considered. I took the two sets of films to the radiologists down the hall. I enjoyed bringing positive x-rays to the specialists to show them I knew what I was doing and because I usually learned something as well. This trip was no exception. I still had not focused on the fact that the pathology I was going to display was my own. . . . When I told them it was me, there was an immediate change in their casual manner. They weighed their words carefully as they examined the radiograph and awkwardly asked me a few questions. The changed demeanor of these friends of mine cut through my clinical dispassion and raised the first red flag in my mind. I felt my initial fear.
>
> By now I was beginning to come to grips with what was happening. That pint-sized cauliflower that I had so recently discovered on a piece of celluloid was in fact a tumor—a cancer. It was living quietly deep within my body. Though I had no knowledge at that point of what kind of cancer it was, its strategic location suggested that it could bring my life to an end at any time. In a space of five minutes it had come out of nowhere to become the focal point of my life, or perhaps the focal point of the rest of my life. . . . The radiologist wanted to take x-rays of my abdomen. The smock he gave me was absurdly short and as I padded down the corridor in my stocking feet with my knees showing I suddenly understood that I was a patient.
>
> As I climbed onto the cold, metallic x-ray table I had reason and time to think about this. The x-ray that the radiologist had scheduled for me was an intravenous pyelogram, which required sequential views of my kidneys over a half-hour

period. During that time I was not to leave the table. Lying on that hospital slab, staring at the maze of electronic equipment over my head on that March morning in 1975, I felt alone and in agony, desperate to talk to someone—the physician I had picked to consult, my wife, my parents, anyone. I was bursting to share the calamity. But all I could do was lie there with my eyes helplessly scanning the gadgetry around the room, looking for some safe harbor from the anxiety that suddenly inundated me [pp. 4–6].

Having diagnosed his own cancer, Mullan slowly moves from the role of physician to that of a cancer patient. With no one to lean on, he is overwhelmed by anxiety.

While most patients respond to the diagnosis with either initial adaptive denial or a shock of agony, some, a very few, face it with humor. In the essay, "A Splendid Day," by 46-year-old housewife Molly Ingle Michie (1980), we see the author accept the diagnosis of her lung cancer ("broncho-alveolar cell carcinoma") with a sense of humor that nonetheless does not deny the threat to her life. Humor provides Michie with the distance she needs to face the threat without being overwhelmed by it.

The surgeon did not pussyfoot around about the likelihood of my dying. He said that half the people with my disease were alive one year after diagnosis. Only three out of a hundred were alive five years later. The night I found out the diagnosis, I scribbled down a list of dreaded tasks that I would never have to do again—

(1) give large dinner parties
(2) clean the oven
(3) scrub floors
(4) wash delicate things by hand
(5) remove stains

The second thing that I did was to get a calendar and try to figure out a convenient time for me to die.

Then I made a list of people who are already dead, people I would enjoy seeing. I drew it up like a list for a cocktail party.

Until my surgeon told me that I was dying, I never cared much for euphemisms. I preferred the word "dying," for instance, to "passing on" or "going to sleep in the Lord." Now, however, I've decided that dying is a word that absolutely requires a euphemism if you're about to do it.

People recoil if I tell them that I'm about to die. They (and I) feel better if I say I'm about to "kick the bucket" or to "check out" or to "bow out." It's not the metaphorical humor of these euphemisms that makes them more acceptable socially. It's rather, I think, that they describe a familiar scene. All of us at some time have kicked a bucket or checked out or bowed out. But none of us has ever died. Moreover, kicking the bucket and checking out and bowing out are positive actions that we have taken cheerfully and vigorously *at a time that suited us.*

Things to be glad about while dying of cancer:

(1) I don't have to worry about getting cancer anymore. (I always expected to get cancer of the foot because of the x-ray machines that we played with in shoe stores when I was a little girl.)

(2) I had a wonderful trip to Jamaica.

(3) I don't have to worry about gray hair. I don't have to worry about rosacea.

There are only two *real benefits.*

(1) I found out that people love me who I would never have guessed love me. I would have died without knowing.

(2) I won't have to learn the metric system [pp. 410–411].

DENIAL OF DIAGNOSIS

Denial, not wanting to know, is the most effective defense of the tumor patient. It first appears after the patient hears the diagnosis; it represents an attempt to deal with the overwhelming shock and is a hedge against the fear that close friends and family will withdraw. Most patients need to employ this kind of denial at least once during the course of their illness. Patients who use denial live, talk, and act as if they did not understand the consequences of their disease. Sometimes they split off the affected part, dealing with it only on a rational plane. Patients who are told the truth about their illness may behave in this way no less often than do patients who are told consoling fictions. Patients who deny behave as if they had a double bookkeeping system.

Simple forms of denial include an overtly optimistic attitude toward the introduction of therapeutic measures. More complicated forms of denial in the initial stage of illness might involve irrational perceptions, such as that the doctor may have made an erroneous diagnosis or the laboratory tests were mixed up. Such denial protects the self of the patient and eases the feelings of disintegration and of losing one's world.

We call this initial denial adaptive denial. It helps the patient deal with the diagnosis and the suggested treatment methods. According to Weisman (1979), such denial is a way of simplifying the complexities of the cancer patient's new life. When one is faced with a threat from which escape is difficult, denial mutes distress, at least temporarily. Weismann asserts, "Denial has three aims: (1) preserving the status quo, (2) simplifying a relationship, and (3) eliminating differences between what was and what will be" (p. 44). Family and treatment team members should understand the function of this form of denial and support it. There is no reason to hinder it.

Initial adaptive denial may have a positive influence on prognosis. Women who three months after mastectomy show adaptive denial also show a strong will to fight the disease. They have a higher survival rate after five years than do women who resign themselves and develop a hopeless-and-helpless syndrome (Greer, Morris, and Pettingale, 1979). Adaptive denial does not mean that patients do not recognize that they are sick. Rather, they adopt an overly positive attitude toward the possible success of treatment. This early, all-inclusive adaptive denial, if supported by good medical guidance, later gives way to a more selective denial, directed only to particular aspects of the disease.

Theo Hosch (1986), a high school student with Hodgkin's disease, describes in detail his intense, long denial during the diagnostic phase:

> Even when I discovered a knot as big as a pea under the skin on the right side of my neck, I didn't suspect anything unpleasant. "Discovered" is not the right word, but I felt it and paid no more attention to it. . . . Because my parents were on vacation I was a bit bored. Looking for some distraction, I got the idea of going to see my doctor. As a reason for my visit I told him that I wanted to know if I would pass the army review. But my first meeting with this doctor, which was only meant to be a visit, developed differently from my expectations. . . .
>
> Our initial friendly relationship would keep its relaxed character for some time but when the doctor started to touch and examine me the mood changed slowly but steadily. After he had carefully examined my neck, armpits and inguinal region, he sat down in his chair again. He told me that something might be wrong; he had seen things like this before. In any case, it had to be checked out and he suggested a chest x-ray. . . . I wasn't in the least impressed by all of this. I was happy to have had some distraction and went home. The next weekend was not influenced by what had happened at my physician's; it was like many other weekends, untroubled and carefree [pp. 16–18].

After the biopsy of the knot, Hosch writes:

> Still I didn't get any unpleasant ideas. What had happened
> was a bit painful and unpleasant, but for me it was not a reason
> to worry. . . . I was still not worried. . . .
> Inexplicably, my parents were not so happy about the
> events. For an adult, a little knot in the neck was probably more
> cause for concern than for an adolescent. . . .
> Slowly, very slowly, my mood too became adequate. But
> there was not the least trace of helplessness or hopelessness
> that one often sees in cancer patients. I forbade the use of the
> word "cancer"; looking back at it, that was the best thing I could
> have done [pp. 20–24].

Hosch's youth may have been partly responsible for the especially strong
denial he exhibited. It is equally likely, however, that his impulse to deny
so strongly was grounded in his sister's death of leukemia some years
earlier.

The East German writer Reimann (1984), a woman in her late 30s,
describes in successive diary entries how a similarly strong attempt to
deny the suspicion of breast cancer only gradually gave way to a
recognition of the seriousness of the diagnosis:

> February 26, 1968
> I lay in bed for physical, but also for psychological reasons,
> because something has grown on me (as Kafka would say)
> which does not really belong to a woman's body—not a baby,
> by any means. I cried each morning while awakening but then
> I worked intensively, because I saw myself already dead, my
> opus unfinished. . . . In the meantime, I have had many medical
> examinations and everything seems to indicate that it is a
> "benign" growth.

> April 4, 1968
> . . . I have to finish my book; maybe it is a race with a
> possibly serious illness.

> July 22, 1968
> Monday I was at Professor S's. I am healthy! I can't tell you
> how happy I was as I walked out of the clinic.

> July 25, 1968
> A weight fell off my heart. Now I only have to sacrifice one
> more day, so Dr. M. can cut out this knot. . . .

> August 8, 1968
> The operation went well but I am in trouble again because
> while cutting they found more knots. Danger might still be

lurking in the "bush"... Dr. M. is sending them to the institute to be examined....

September 10, 1968

Only a few lines—after a long silence. Today I got the verdict for which I had been waiting for months and for which I was, in some way, ready. I have cancer. . . . Keep your fingers crossed for me. I am scared. I would like to be a hero, but I'm not.

September 19, 1968

You shouldn't think it's too bad. Since I went to the doctor in time, the growth hasn't spread yet and there is no immediate life threat. Naturally, it is revolting to be cut in half like that. This morning I cried a whole lot, but now I am calmer [pp. 273-284].

Although she denied her suspicions of cancer, Reimann was unconsciously aware of it long before test results got back from the laboratory. Strong initial adaptive denial can be seen in the writings of many cancer authors. Denial occurs in all phases of the illness, but is strongest the first few days after the diagnosis has been received (Weisman, 1972; Lipowski, 1979; Lazarus, 1981).

In the diagnostic and initial treatment phase, the relationship between doctor and patient can be disrupted if the doctor is not sufficiently sensitive to the patient's needs for information. An overly anxious doctor may equivocate, behavior that only leads to confusion. Patients also infer a great deal from silence and from uncharacteristic behavior, as we saw in Rollin's (1976) account of her initial interview. The disruption of open communication between doctor and patient can adversely influence the course of the illness, the way a patient responds to treatment, and the patient's psychosocial balance.

Both in this early phase and later, the patient is very sensitive to the behavior of others and quickly senses if the doctor and members of the family avoid answering his questions or try to lull his fears with unconfirmed hope. Such avoidance tactics further weaken the feelings of self that have already been threatened by the diagnosis, and contribute to the patient's inner retreat, thus fostering a depressive state. A patient who feels disappointed by his doctors in this first phase of the illness will be overwhelmed by fear and despair in later phases. He will avoid approaching his doctors in times of need and his inner isolation will only increase. If the support of family members and friends is also missing, the patient is doomed to die a "social death" before physical death occurs (Cassileth and Cassileth, 1982). As Weisman (1979) puts it, the ideal strategy is candor together with hope, tact, compassion, common sense, and straightforward statements. These are safeguards against platitudes, circumlocutions, apologies, and irrelevancies.

Alsop (1973) indicates the importance to the cancer patient of honest, empathic communication on the part of the physician during the diagnostic phase. The trust that was established between Alsop and his doctor, John Glick, at the early stage immensely helped the patient to deal with the constant threat of death over a long period of time:

> That first day, John Glick was very impersonal and professional, but I liked him instinctively, and so did Tish. Later, liking grew into affection and admiration and also into genuine friendship, a relationship not easily attained between a 28-year-old and a man twice his age.
>
> Dr. Glick had asthma as a boy (as I did), and he has the slightly hunched shoulders of many asthmatics. He has a thin, sallow, interesting, and obviously intelligent face, and a certain unselfconscious intensity of manner. He has a good sense of humor, but when he is chasing after clues on which to base a diagnosis, he has the humorless intensity of a bloodhound on the trail. Even that first day, it seemed to me that he was genuinely interested in my case, perhaps in part for the same reason that Sherlock Holmes, after a long diet of easy solutions, would find a really difficult case so stimulating that he felt no need of his usual dose of laudanum [pp. 26-27]

Such interested candor is not always easy for the physician, as Alsop would later learn.

Sometimes the denial of the full import of the diagnosis is quite conscious, as can be seen from the following passage from Alsop. After receiving the diagnosis of cancer, the patient must deal with the question raised by his treatments. Along with his doctor he must weigh the possibility of a cure or of an arrest of the illness, on one hand, against the painful side effects and the change in quality of life on the other. And all this must be weighed in the context of an altered view of mortality.

> Would it really be worthwhile to spend a month or more cooped up all alone in a laminar flow room, losing my hair and my flesh, either to die in the room or to emerge a bald skeleton and wait for death? Would it not be more sensible to reach for Hamlet's "Bare bodkin," in the shape of a bottle of sleeping pills? And then a sense of the reality of death crowded in on me—the end of a pleasant life, never to see Tish or Andrew or Nicky or the four older children again, never to go to Needwood again, or laugh with friends, or see the spring come. There came upon me a terrible sense of aloneness, of vulnerability, of nakedness, of helplessness. I got up, and fumbled in

my shaving kit, and found another sleeping pill, and at last dozed off. . . .

I never again had a night as bad as that night, nor, I think, shall I ever again. For a kind of protective mechanism took over, after the first shock of being told of the imminence of death, and I suspect that this is true of most people. Partly, this is a perfectly conscious act of will—a decision to allot to the grim future only its share of your thoughts and no more....

The conscious effort to close off one's mind, or part of it, to the inevitability of death plays a part, I suspect, in the oddly cheerful tone of much of what I've written in this book [pp. 30–31].

4

PSYCHOLOGICAL REACTIONS
TO THE
INITIATION OF TREATMENT

If I would have agreed to an operation, I would have become a patient. I would have definitely stepped into the role of a patient. This way I am not a patient, not healthy, terminally sick, but not a patient. Till the end I will be able to "play" the role of a healthy and normal person. It is not really "play" but a distinction between two forms of existence. I still believe that I have chosen correctly [Noll, 1984, pp. 123–124].

Because cancer forms a large group of diseases of varying incidence, site, anatomical extent, pathology, clinical course, and prognosis, it is amenable to surgery, responds to ionizing radiation, and can be treated by chemical agents and hormones. This variability of intrinsic features and therefore of diagnostic and treatment methods encourages the use of a multimodal, collective, team approach. Aggressive multimodal therapy typically consists of radical resection of all gross tumors wherever possible, followed by radiation therapy to eradicate any remaining disease at the primary site and by continued chemotherapy for any residual disease elsewhere in the body.

But all these methods of oncological treatment—surgery, radiation, and chemotherapy—have an intrusive, aggressive character and are rightfully feared by patients because of their unpleasant side- and aftereffects. One frequently hears from doctors and patients alike that the treatment is worse than the disease. Descriptions of cancer therapy are drawn from the language of warfare: The patient's body is "under attack" or "invaded", as Sontag (1977, p. 84) notes and the only treatment is "counterattack." Cancer cells do not simply multiply, but are "invasive"; they first set up tiny "outposts" (micrometastases) and "colonize" from the original tumor. In radiation therapy the metaphors are taken from aerial warfare: patients' tumors are "bombarded" with toxic rays. In chemotherapy, words from chemical warfare are used, for example, "poison." Treatment aims at "killing" the cancer cells without killing the patient (Sontag, 1977, p. 65). Patients fear that they have passively surrendered to unknown and potentially destructive powers. That intrusive treatments are often not delivered by the patient's primary physician exacerbates this fear of the unknown (Meerwein, 1985).

Military metaphors abound in the poem "Bulletins from a War" by Helen Webster (1980), an American poet who suffered from breast cancer:

Bulletins From a War

Civil war. My body is
the battleground.
Left breast falls first.
One lumpy legion conceals
treacherous intent.
Occupied territory:
The lymph system.
Suspected of abetting
the enemy,
ovaries are sacrificed.
Five-year cease fire
follows.
Traitors, adrenal glands
fall to a cutting attack.
Uneasy truce ensues.
Stealthily sternum, ribs,
vertebrae are invaded.
Chemical warfare
routs violators.
Lymph zone demilitarized.
Hostile forces encroach
into abdominal cavity.
Disposal system blockaded.
Shock troops counterattack:
Unleash a new biological
weapon.
Establish alternate route

through the colon.
Armies deadlocked.
Campaign succeeds brilliantly, briefly.
Hostile forces regroup
at previous battle site.
Raiding parties partly
shut down essential services.
Cut again.
Reroute again.
Lethal chemicals
poison the enemy.
Among the casualties:
innocent bystanders.
Hair falls.
Mucous membranes massacred.
White blood cells slaughtered.
Current report:
State of siege.
                              —Webster (1980, p. 35)

SURGERY

For centuries surgery was the only method of treating cancer, and it is still the major form of treatment today for the vast majority (75-80%) of curable patients (Sherman et al.; 1987). The modern cancer operation consists of a wide excision of the primary tumor and its direct extensions and the removal of the regional lymph nodes when appropriate. Oncologists differentiate between curative surgery, localized to the tissue of origin and its regional draining lymph nodes; preventive surgery, the preferred treatment for premalignant lesions; diagnostic surgery, or biopsy, often done during an exploratory operation; palliative surgery, to cure or prevent symptoms and to enhance comfort and prolong life; reductive surgery, where one removes only the bulk of the tumor in the hope that chemotherapy, radiation therapy, or both may contain or cure the remaining tumor; and surgery for recurrences of cancer and relief of pain.

If the surgical intervention is not connected with disfigurement or the loss of a body part, then surgery is considered the optimal treatment method. The intense fears that are common prior to the operation are usually quickly dispelled with the success of this type of surgery.

Amputations, which attack the patient's physical integrity, especially organs or body parts that are strongly connected to sex-specific roles and thus define the patient's identity and self-worth, can bring with them postoperative depression or even psychotic decompensation. For amputee patients, the operation is the real drama; the cancer itself and the threat of death become less significant compared with the immediate threat of destruction of their physical and psychological integrity. The younger the patient, the more intense the reaction, since in youth the feeling of self-worth is strongly connected with external appearance. In his novel *Cancer Ward*, Solzhenitsyn (1968), a cancer survivor himself, has Anya, an 18-year-old girl with breast cancer question Demka, an adolescent boy facing surgery for a bone tumor in his leg:

> "What do you mean, cut your leg off? Are they crazy? Or don't they want to bother curing you? Don't let them do it. Better die than live without a leg. What sort of life is the life of a cripple? Life has to be enjoyed."
>
> Yes, of course, she was right again. What was life with a crutch? Suppose he was sitting next to her, what would he do with his crutches? And what would it be like with a stump? No. Life without a leg was no life at all [p. 98].

In a moving scene later in the novel, Anya comes to Demka in tears and panic:

> She was wailing into the pillow.
> "Please, Assenka! Tell me what it is. Tell me."
> But he had almost guessed.
> "They'll am-pu-tate!"
> She wept and wept. Then she moaned:
> "Oo-o-o!"
> Demka could not remember ever hearing such a wail of grief as this terrible "O-o-o!" . . .
> For the first time Demka saw her wet, red, blotched, pitiful and angered face. "Who wants a woman with one breast? Who? At seventeen!" she screamed at him as though it were all his fault.
> "How will I go to the beach?" she wailed, as this fresh thought stabbed her. "The beach! How will I go swimming?" The idea twisted through her like a corkscrew, pierced her and flung her away from Demka and down to the floor, where her body collapsed and she clutched her head in her hands.
> Finally she demands that he kiss her cancerous breast and asks, "Will you remember it? You will remember that I had it, won't you? And what it was like?"

She did not remove it, she did not move away; he returned to the brown nipple, and his lips gently did what her future baby would never be able to do at this breast. No one entered, and he went on kissing the marvel that hung above him.

Today a marvel, tomorrow into the basket [p. 82].

Alan Stoudemire (1983), the young physician who developed a malignant fibrous histiocytoma of the right tibia during his psychiatric residency, describes his emotional reaction to the amputation of his leg. In describing his feelings, Stoudemire borrows from the work of Pollock, who identified the various components of acute mourning:

> Following the amputation and an initial phase of shocked disbelief, my reaction to the loss of the limb was one of intense grief similar to the experience of losing a loved, valued, and highly cathected object. This phase of my grief paralleled the "acute state of mourning" that Pollock . . . described as consisting of shock, grief, pain, separation anxiety and anger, and the gradual process of decathexis of the lost object. For myself, this process involved not only the leg as the lost object but also a lost image of myself.
>
> My emotional states fluctuated. At times I certainly was morbidly depressed, but perhaps the predominant affect I felt was anger: a painful, lonely, helpless, diffuse rage:
>
> As the shock, grief, pain, and anger abated, I gradually shifted to a "chronic mourning stage" in which all of the adaptive capabilities of the ego are summoned to come to grips with the reality of the loss, and the necessity of making an adaptation to that reality. In this adaptive phase, the ego begins to integrate the loss into a new self-image and to adjust to the demands of reality [p. 380].

Still following Pollock, Stoudemire goes on to identify the special role of anger in mourning reaction:

> When there is anger about the loss, it is indicative that the separation is recognized and acknowledged. In this sense anger is restitutive, as cathexis is discharged through the affective experience of anger. Thus, the anger is in the service of the mastery of shock, panic and grief. As to the reasons for the anger, we must recognize that the rage is a narcissistic rage. It is as if the child is screaming, "It happens to me and I have no control over it!" When the rage is discharged diffusely, frustra-

tion at being left is avoided, as is the feeling of helplessness
[p. 351].

Patients whose bodies are mutilated by operations such as a
mastectomy or the amputation of a limb need psychological support to
face the painful perception of the change in their body. Mastectomy
threatens the sexual self-image of the woman, and the lessening of her
sexual and physical attractiveness can bring about self-devaluation and an
identity crisis. The same is true for operations that affect procreative
ability or the libido, such as operations on the testicles or ovaries.

Losing a part of the body or being mutilated is always connected to
a depressive afterreaction. The reaction might appear immediately after
the operation or remain latent for several weeks. It is important to make
patients aware that depression is a normal reaction and to suggest possible
ways of dealing with these strong feelings. The loss of a body part or a
body function requires a period of mourning similar to that felt after the
loss of someone close, as we saw in Stoudemire's description.

For some patients, the only way to deal with the loss is by finding an
outside aggressor onto whom they can project their intense rage at having
lost a part of themselves. The doctor is a ready target. The expression of
these resentments should not unduly upset the doctor. At the very least,
they indicate that the patient is still interested in living and functioning. If
patients feel free to express their rage, they are better able to resolve it
than if they turn the rage against themselves and become depressed.

Smaller operations, or operations on less emotionally loaded internal
organs, are generally less problematic for patients and do not provoke
such strong emotional reactions. The success of these operations is
apparent almost immediately afterward, when the patient begins to realize
that the malignant tumor has been removed by the knife. Until the precise
histological results are received, patients are still anxious, but they realize
that the most important indications of the success of an operation are the
postoperative signs, such as wound healing, gaining strength, and so on.
That is why patients often talk extensively about their physical recovery
and the very day after the operation rush to tell their doctors that they feel
physically fit. A rapid recovery somehow seems to be the magic proof that
the illness was not so serious after all.

Still, cancer surgery on any body part, external or internal, is always
initially approached with a great deal of fear and gives rise to frightening
fantasies. Diggelmann (1979) conveys how the overwhelming fear of a
second operation (following earlier brain surgery) totally overcomes him
and leads to an all-encompassing fear of death:

December 7th, 1978.
The dice have fallen; the histologist declared the verdict.

They found out that in the right flap of my lung a tumor is building its nest, a malignant one.

... What good does it do me that the specialist tells me that my lungs are so big that even if two thirds were cut away I could still live very well with the rest. That's not the point. The point is that another piece of my life is being taken away and I don't know why or what for. I don't know what crime I committed. I have to admit that a deep depression has overtaken me in the last few days.

... Depression: more accurately, it is fear. An incredible fear that cannot be put into words, even though as a writer I should be able to handle words. It is a fundamental fear, diffuse fear. I am afraid of myself. I am afraid of my surroundings. I am afraid of everything that there is no reason to fear. I am not afraid of the operation, nor the anaesthesia. I don't think of it. ... But the fear they can't take from me [pp. 49-50].

The East German writer Maxi Wander (1980), feeling out of control, dependent, and forced to surrender to unknown forces, sees her anaesthetist as death:

In my semi-sleep the anaesthetist appears ... that's the one who will put me to sleep. He is truly "death" for me. My thoughts become confused under the influence of the Dormuti [medicine]. Unconscious, and at the mercy of so many white coats in the operating room, how can one not be afraid? [p. 16].

Stoudemire (1983) similarly describes his final memory prior to the amputation of his leg as a fantasy of death:

A final memory: Prior to the amputation, the anesthesiologist was putting in the intravenous line. I heard the metal instruments clattering; knives, I fantasized. I had never really asked how they were going to cut it off. The anesthesia mask made me feel as if I were going to be suffocated to death. I tried to pull it off, but my hands were restrained. The last thing I recall was one nurse saying to another, "This will just be a short case." A short case!! [p. 381].

In the terror of a threatening cancer operation, the patient often tries to hold on to any available support. This is what the Swiss author Maya

Beutler (1980) does. First she tries to recover her good internal object, her father, who survived a neck operation similar to the one she is about to undergo before he finally died of his tumor at the age of 79:

> "You are my beloved child," you [her father] told me on the eve of your operation. Tonight I turned this sentence around in my head. My ears buzzed, "You are my beloved child, you are my beloved child." Like a marble this statement rolls back and forth. . . .
> . . . Tomorrow morning I will be operated on. . . . Father, now I could talk to you, now I could hug you, everything has its right time. . . . Now I am on your side and let the typewriter rattle "you are my beloved child," then it has to become ten to eight for the children, that's all that matters, they want to go to work, to school, and I have to let them go, to step back, I want, that's why I rattle, that they can hear it clearly through the closed door, and will sigh relieved: "At least she is writing, she can forget it a little." I want them to be consoled [pp. 55–56].

Then Beutler turned also to the comforting support of her faith in God, which developed when she was a child and is connected to her beloved father. The following passage is addressed to her son:

> I once asked your grandfather "How big is God?" and he looked up from his paper over the rim of his glasses and said, "Unimaginable, I mean: he is entirely unimaginable." I ran into the garden and laid down on my back and imagined him anyway: God is as big as the cloud over the roof, no, as big as the sky over the garden, no, over the city, no, like the sky over the fields, no, behind the wood behind the mountains, no, no. I suddenly started to cry, out of fear of this size. I went back into the house and father folded his paper . . . . "Maybe you understand it now," he said, "What one can't imagine one has to endure." I can endure it, we all will endure it I am sure. Life is unimaginable, life is insecure, always. You taught me that from the very first" [p. 74].

The more the surgeon understands the preoperative cancer patient's acute fears and needs, the better. Although no amount of understanding will entirely counter the terrors of death or the horror of an amputated limb, the surgeon's getting to know the patient, his readiness to listen to the patient's anxieties, and his willingness to extend empathy and support can go a long way to alleviate the dread.

POSTOPERATIVE PHASE

The main psychological threats at this stage are, initially, the loss of control associated with the anesthesia and the physical aftereffects of the surgery, and, then, more deeply, the dawning perception that part of one's body has been irrevocably cut off.

Maya Beutler's inability to move her tongue, talk, or drink adds to her almost incoherent and conflict-filled fantasies of her dead father and to her sense of her own incapacity:

> Father, who are you—why do you call? My mouth is full of rocks, I can't move them, but I have to emphasize: Here I am, I know for sure this is me, I move myself, I brace myself against the mountains. . . . I have to turn these mountains around. No: Stones, doesn't one say stones instead of bread, did mother say it? I still wait for bread from you and you give me stones? . . . I now understand everything. Now they wall me up: Yes, I hear, I see. . . . To press the stones till water is flowing. Why did everything dry up, the desert? Here I am father, I push against these rocks, I would like to move the mountains, time, I want to get up, I want. . . . Suddenly I am a woman, I push and press and a tiny piece of wet life can shoot out, if I just continue pressing. "Thanks for everything." Do children fall out of one's mouth? Who put concrete in here? Open up! I am knocking, open up [pp. 78–79].

Beutler's rage intensifies when she regains full consciousness and finds herself still unable to speak or move. Extremely upset, she pulls out her intravenous tubes and becomes even more upset when her doctor offers her an injection in an attempt to calm her. She lashes out like a sassy child:

> Injection? Against dynamite, does this help these days? I know what they want to give me. The old kind of life, no thanks, no, no, that's the wrong way, the entire direction is wrong. I'll take myself a whole new life. I'll take it with my thumb and forefinger [p. 84].

Diggelmann's (1979) fantasies also go wild as he lies in the intensive care unit after his lung operation, but as normal consciousness returns he becomes increasingly aware of his pain—both physical and psychological:

I spent last night in intensive care; it was horrible. Tortured by pain and nightmares. Every time one thought one would wake up and woke up, the air and night were filled with vicious ill-natured tumors. One recognized them, and one didn't. One couldn't make sense of them. They didn't belong there, but they did. Finally this night too ended. . . .

They push some kind of button and immediately strange yellow-white lines begin to move on the monitor. Maybe they are little monsters sitting on rays sweeping over the monitor?

I slowly understand why this is called the intensive care unit. It is the core, the nucleus, of all agony a human being can suffer, being caught in a circle. . . . Hell is, that you start to accept everything, against your will because you tell yourself: You didn't do anything wrong. You should have taken care earlier and you shouldn't have come here in the first place. Now you are here [pp. 63–64].

The pressures toward denial are as strong in the postoperative stage as they are in the diagnostic phase of cancer. Though in the first days after an operation, denial may once again serve an adaptive function in getting the patient back on his feet, it is obviously untenable as a long-term response to the loss that is involved. Nor, with the physical evidence of the loss so readily apparent, is it really possible to suppress the emotional reaction indefinitely as we see in Betty Rollin's (1976) account of her denial—encouraged by both her visitors and her doctor—right after her mastectomy. Rollin was only superficially able to fend off the strong feelings provoked by the loss of her breast:

I got many congratulations for being so brave and cheerful. I liked that, so I got more brave and more cheerful. And the more brave and cheerful I was, the more everyone seemed to love me, so I kept it up. I became positively euphoric. . . .

But when I did think or talk about it, the Glad Girl kept shining through: I'm glad I only lost one breast instead of two; I'm glad I was sort of flat-chested to start with, so it won't look all that much different; I'm glad it doesn't hurt much (no doubt about it, a good dose of pain and Pollyanna would have closed out of town); I'm glad it won't show when I'm dressed, say the way an arm or a leg or a nose would; and oh, yes, I'm glad I'm not dead and—well, who needs a breast anyway, you can't do anything with a breast, you can't type with it or walk on it or play "Melancholy Baby" with it? And besides all that, a breast is something you have two of, so if it serves a purpose (I did remember vaguely that it figured in sex) there's still the other one. . . . I wanted to (and did) believe and hear everything that was nice. If, conversely, it wasn't nice, I didn't believe it, didn't hear it, and I certainly didn't think about it. Not yet. . . .

While I was in the hospital I almost never used the word "breast," it was tit this and tit that.

Rough-tough talk was not only part of my increasingly agile defense, it was also another good crowd-pleaser. Whatta girl, I'd hear them think. Whatta sensa humor. What guts. . . .

Singermann [the surgeon] also congratulated me for having such a good-looking wound and for healing so nicely. (I suppose he was really congratulating himself, but I didn't read it that way at the time.) As far as having an attractive wound, I had to take his word for it, because I wasn't about to look. Most of the time, I couldn't look because I was bandaged. When he changed the bandage I could have looked, but I didn't. I was not even tempted. I'd sit on the edge of my bed and he'd unwrap me and we'd yammer away in our usual language (tit, shit, fuck, et al.) and I would pick a dirt spot on the window and, as more of the wrapping came off, I'd stare harder and harder at the spot. I knew what I was doing. I knew that one look might blow my whole act, and I wasn't going to do that. My act was all I had [pp. 71–78].

Together with the patient, Rollin's surgeon kept up his denial, thus standing in the way of her dealing with her loss.

Lorde (1980) also describes the futility of her attempts to continue to deny her feelings as the pain she feels in the breast that she no longer has brings home her loss more cruelly. At first, her denial shielded her:

That next day after the operation was an incredible high. I now think of it as the euphoria of the second day. The pain was minimal. I was alive. The sun was shining. I remember feeling a little simple but rather relieved it was all over, or so I thought. I stuck a flower in my hair and thought "This is not as bad as I was afraid of."

From time to time I would put my hand upon the flattish mound of bandages on the right side of my chest and say to myself—my right breast is gone, and I would shed a few tears if I was alone. But I had no real emotional contact yet with the reality of the loss; it was as if I had been emotionally anesthetized also, or as if the only feelings I could reach were physical ones, and the scar was not only hidden under bandages but as yet was feeling little pain. When I looked at myself in the mirror even, the difference was not at all striking, because of the bulkiness of the bandages [pp. 36-37].

But, then, pain arose that could not be blocked out:

My breast which was no longer there would hurt as if it were being squeezed in a vise. That was perhaps the worst pain of all, because it would come with a full complement of horror that I was to be reminded of my loss by suffering in a part of me which was no longer there. I suddenly seemed to get weaker rather than stronger. The euphoria and numbing effects of the anesthesia were beginning to subside [p. 38].

In those two instances, the denial was actively encouraged by the patient's doctor. Cheerful patients are easier to deal with; they flatter their doctors' expertise and tactfully help them to suppress their own fears of cancer. However, as the following journal entries by Maxi Wander (1980) show, the physician's need to deny can be quite intolerable to the patient, who is all too aware of what has been irrevocably cut off. Wander's doctor's refusal to answer her questions increased her fears. His self-protective distance, as well as that of the nurses, came across as coldness and lack of concern. The end result was that this otherwise optimistic patient became deeply depressed, bemoaning her isolation and dwelling on her death. In time, she came to believe that her doctor's behavior was impeding her recovery:

Friday, September 10th
4 a.m. already. The thermometer. Today I am calm and have no temperature. Blood tests over and over again. Seven o'clock the first doctor's visit, eight o'clock the second visit, eight doctors, six men, two women and two nurses. Scary! They only look at the chart at the foot of the bed. The person doesn't interest them? What person is this? Who is lying here? But they are interested only in the tumor [p. 13]

Friday, September 17th
What the doctors communicated over the next few days was not only cancer—that seems to be beyond a doubt anyway—but also that they didn't catch all of it. I can gather this from the laconic statements that slowly but surely are extracted from them. I punch holes in them with my questions. Maybe other patients are resigned to their fate. Why don't they

look at people? Why can't they explain things better to the patient. In vain I wait for consolation, for someone to come and say "You've been having a hard time, but it's over now!" [p. 19].

She continues writing:

Nothing! I am left by myself, with my destroyed body and my brain which does not stop thinking. "You have to breathe deeply", says the nurse, "otherwise you will get pneumonia!" But I can't breathe deeply. It hurts my stomach, every breath hurts. And I breathe and think of Hugo who was redeemed by his pneumonia.

But to die so suddenly, without finishing bringing up Dani [son]? Vain enough to think who might mourn me. Not for a long time, anyway. Soon I will be forgotten.

Who will sit down on my bed?   [pp. 20–21].

She goes on:

Saturday, September 18th

Christiana, the nurse, while changing the dressing: "Don't look." But I did look. A thick red cut across my chest to the armpit. Maybe I am too weak to be scared. I am like a wounded animal that plays dead so as not to be hurt again [p. 23]

Wander continues to write in her journal:

. . . I can't bear it here any longer without a doctor one can latch onto. Here everything is anonymous: the patients and the doctors. An atmosphere in which I can't become healthy [p. 24].

This negative example shows us how important it is for the patient in the postoperative phase to feel that her surgeon and treatment team are supportive and caring. The more psychologically contained patients can feel in the hospital environment, the faster will be their physical recovery and their regaining hope for the future.

RADIATION THERAPY

Radiation therapy consists of the therapeutic use of ionizing radiation, such as x-rays, gamma-rays, or electrons, for the treatment of malignancies. The use of ionizing radiation in medicine stems from Roentgen's discovery of x-rays in 1895 and Curie's discovery of radium in 1898 (Sherman et al., 1987). External radiation uses orthovoltage ray generators, linear accelerators, betatrons, telecobalt, and telecaesium machines. The area and depth of the target must be precisely defined by means of preliminary radiographs and sometimes by LT scans to ensure that the radiation field will exactly encompass the tumor. The patient must be precisely positioned so that the treatment can be reproduced on a daily basis. The treatment team is composed of a radiation oncologist, a physicist, a dosimetrist, a maintenance engineer, and technicians. With the help of a computer simulator, x-ray machines are employed to select and double-check the appropriate field. Radiotherapy can be used either as a method of cure or as a palliative, for example to prolong a symptom-free period or to relieve distressing symptoms, such as pain or hemorrhage.

Seventy to eighty percent of all cancer patients undergo radiation therapy. The need for radiation therapy signals to the patient that an operation was not entirely successful or that the cancer has spread.

Radiation therapy is pervaded by mystery and "inhuman" fantasies; it makes the patient uneasy and uncomfortable. Beutler (1980) describes how radiation therapy made her feel a stranger to herself:

> When my hands touch, they recoil. My brittleness scares me, I reject myself . . . dried up and tired, I would like to put a permanent membrane of sleep between myself and me, I am day after day, filled up with strangeness, David against Goliath, fifty seven blinded seconds are flung at me at the speed of light [p. 98].

During the treatment, patients cannot see, hear, smell, or feel what is happening as they lie under the huge cobalt machine. They are left alone with outlines drawn on their skin, indicating the exact place on the body where the rays are being shot, and are given orders by a voice through a microphone behind a glass door.

In this situation, which can readily foster paranoid fears and reactions, it is especially important to inform the patient of exactly what to expect during the treatment and the duration of each treatment period. The patient should be carefully informed of side effects, such as anorexia, nausea, dizziness, tiredness, vomiting, diarrhea or constipation, and skin irritation at the site of the therapy. It is necessary to explain to the patient, sensitively and empathically, that though radiation therapy destroys the healthy cells as well as the pathological cells, the healthy cells recover quickly and will soon begin to function normally.

The waiting rooms outside radiation units often elevate patients' anxieties. Left in strange surroundings with people who may be very ill, patients can easily be overcome by fears of isolation and annihilation. The waiting rooms are often dark, since they tend to be located in the basement of the hospital, and are highly technical in appearance and rigidly organized. Frequently, the technician who actually applies the treatment knows virtually nothing about the patient other than how many rays must be applied to what part of his or her body. This adds to the patient's feelings of depersonalization, and the daily confrontation with the other patients sitting anxiously in the waiting room can escalate a patient's fear into despair. As she opens the door of her dressing cabin in the radiotherapy station and looks at the waiting room area, Beutler (1980) thinks:

> I open up the door. Here they are squatting, the heavenly hosts with their plucked feathers. Fischer [another patient] is smiling at me, his hair fluffy and thin. . . . In his blue and white striped morning coat he looks like a dressed up giant in a fairy tale . . . [pp. 98–99].

The impersonal, uncaring attitude of the typical young radiation technicians, who are often unaware of their patients' well-founded fears, can augment those fears and may even precipitate feelings of profound depersonalization. Beutler describes this sense of depersonalization and the sense of isolation it fosters:

> He [Fisher, the patient] is afraid, like I am. He is cold down here, like me. Next please, next please, please don't enter, please enter now, please get on the bed immediately, please don't stall, please let me help you, please move precisely, please, here the millimeter count, today you receive 150 units, tomorrow more, please get used to it, it's manageable isn't it? or why don't you? pain, fear? You can't feel the rays, you can't see them, all guarded by cylinders, what do you imagine? What do you think. Only eight square centimeters are open, we move in pendulum motions . . . [p. 101].

The platitudes of the distant and impersonal staff are of little help as Beutler lies overwhelmed by the side effects of the radiotherapy:

> Ice cold milk, ice cold cream, the nurse maintains, butter put out the fire, to brush with Bepanthen, to sleep with Rohypnol, to endure with Novalgin, I am constantly cold, I am cold, please take me in your arms . . . [p. 104].

What she needs is warmth, which she finds in a fellow patient, not the treatment team:

> Mouse alone, I am mouse alone, we have to move closer together, to warm each other. Curious how Fischer [another patient] uses the words, like "soil on my fields," his sentences are old and dusty, they are rumpled by the wind, but I can feel the warmth: "It actually helps" [p. 113].

Writer Shirley Sikes (1988), who underwent radiation therapy for breast cancer, describes the same feeling of being controlled and left at the mercy of a huge, one-eyed machine:

> When I was irradiated, a giant machine opened its shutter like a malevolent eye. Suspended above me, it seemed to wink closed. It seemed to have an enormous secret.
> When the technicians came back into the room (no danger they said, yet they always returned to their lead-filled walls) they turned me to another position. I felt like a doll being placed on a sill.
> The Cyclops eye rolled open, rolled shut.
> Someone once said, "In the great acts of life, we are alone." [p. 82].

Brigitte Reimann (1984) tries to regain control by counteracting her fear with alcohol. At the same time, the radiation therapy again undermines her denial:

> With the help of a great amount of cognac I get over the radiation pretty well. The first time I was very afraid lying under this cobalt bomb. It was as comfortable as in an inquisition cellar, doctor and physicists with lead aprons, while I was lying naked, exposed to the shooting . . . sometimes I think that I really have cancer or a similar monstrosity . . . [p. 321].

The fear evoked by the life threat and increased by the mysterious quality of the radiation therapy, the impersonality of the treatment team, and the patient's sense of isolation may all coalesce, at this stage, into a powerful, diffuse rage directed alternately at the treatment team and, in some patients, against themselves. Michie describes how her anger, which she personifies as an imaginary bird of prey named A.F. (for Albino Falcon, or Anger Free Floating), would strike out indiscriminantly at everyone she encountered. Michie might prefer her term "free floating anger" over the familiar term "free floating anxiety."

> Into the room came a small, oriental man. A.F. attacked immediately, sinking his pink talons into Dr. Meng L. Lim's yellow neck. World War II lasted from my ninth to my 13th year. Every Saturday afternoon during that time I went with my friends to war movies. We ate popcorn and watched Japs torture heroic American pilots. I developed a hatred and fear of the Japanese. Here was Dr. Lim—Japanese and a radiotherapist. Already he was talking about how many rads he would need to give me to stop the cancer's growth. Already his fingers were looking for evidence of new growth. With his yellow, torturer's mind, I knew he was hoping to find new growth.
>
> I began asking him questions to which I probably did not really want to know the answers. I had refrained from asking them of my surgeon, Ivan Crosby, partly because I didn't want to know and partly because I like him so much and because he obviously hated to give me bad news. I asked him once during the weekend if my kind of cancer was possibly—hopefully— finicky, liking to eat only pleura exclusively. He shook his head sadly and said, "It's not very finicky. It likes other things, too." I did not ask Ivan which other things.
>
> I did ask Dr. Lim immediately. He would enjoy giving me bad news. "If the cancer spreads," he said, "it will most likely go to your liver or to your brain." He told me to come back in one week to be marked for radiation treatments on the linear accelerator. An orderly came to wheel me back to my room.
>
> A.F. let go of Dr. Lim's neck and settled himself on the back of the wheelchair, licking his talons, obviously calmer than before. I felt calmer, too. Some of my anger had found a target. As we were wheeled down the long hall of the radiation oncology department, I began to notice other defects that could absorb some of my anger. The Dutch therapist [radiation technician] waved a cheerful goodbye. She was going to make things difficult for A.F., and me, but we would prevail by ignoring her . . . [p. 417].

The rest of the treatment team gave Michie and A.F. more than enough opportunity:

> Mark-up on Monday was a nightmare for me. I lay on a hard table, in an incredibly uncomfortable position for someone

who had just had a thoracotomy, while pretty, cheerful technicians x-rayed me repeatedly and drew on me with purple magic markers. They would decide that my spine was not exactly straight, move me ever so slightly, and x-ray again. I begged for lead blankets to cover my vulnerable right lung and liver, but they giggled and said there were no lead blankets in radiation oncology. "After all," said one technician, "you are scheduled for 4000 rads. From these little x-rays you get only a few millirads." A.F. clawed her lovely cheeks. . . .

Treatments began the next day. The linear accelerator looks like a machine from Star Wars. I got on its one outstretched arm, my back resting on an open plastic grid. When I was lying comfortably, the arm would move under the machine itself. Technicians would line up my marks with a pattern on the machine above. Computer lights would flash. The technicians would leave the room. A high pitched sound would begin and last for about 15 seconds. The technicians would return, punch a button, the whole machine would revolve 180 degrees, and I would be zapped through the back for 15 seconds. Then the arm would swing me out again and I would dismount. The technicians were all young and beautiful, cheerful and friendly. They chatted with me and with each other. I was convinced that they chatted and drank coffee while they zapped me, and that whether I was zapped for 15 seconds or 25 depended on the whim of three silly 19-year-olds. A.F. got them all.

The next day Dr. Constable himself came in the treatment room to check the set-up. He waited for me outside. Then he showed me how the machine's timing was locked into a computer—how warning bells would ring if anything started to go wrong. How a computer printout recorded every rad and every second. Murphy's Law could not apply to this machine. Nothing could go wrong. A.F. gave him one good scratch for not telling me that the day before.

When later I was in position on the linear accelerator arm, this chaplain appeared. I was somewhat startled, since I was nude to the waist and unaccustomed to being visited by clergy while unattired. When my marks and their pattern were lined up to their satisfaction the technicians left. The chaplain stayed behind a moment, patted me on the arm comfortingly and said, "Remember, we're with you all the way." Then she left.

Tears of anger streamed down my cheek. "You're not with me," I wanted to scream, "If you've got any sense, you and all those pretty technicians are behind thick lead shields. There's no one in here being sizzled but me." A.F. shredded her into bite-size pieces [pp. 419–420].

That the radiation therapy was for the patient's own good and that her anger was "unfair" are beside the point. The passage conveys the rage that many cancer patients, already precariously balanced emotionally, feel as they perceive their bodies bombarded by invisible rays and their movements controlled by others. The passage conveys, too, cancer patients' sensitivity both to intrusions on their privacy, however well meant, and to the hypocrisy of superficial friendliness. Eventually, detailed technical information from her doctor and the establishment of empathic relationships by some of the staff enabled Michie to regain some of her emotional equilibrium. Had they preceded the treatment, the information and empathy might have mitigated some of her fear and anger.

As with cancer surgery, once patients perceive the benefits of radiation treatment, they approach it—and the technicians who apply it—more positively. As Reimann (1984) says, "I can tell you something nice; the radiation helps, there is less pain" (p. 338).

CHEMOTHERAPY

The usefulness of chemotherapy in cancer treatment is well established, with 40 drugs now in active use. Drugs are often used with other therapeutic modalities such as surgery and radiation.

The side effects of chemotherapy are a major limiting factor in their use. These include the interruption of daily life and work, nausea, vomiting, and alopecia (hair loss). Many of the drugs in use can damage the bone marrow and thus the immune system, with consequent infections. They may also affect the endocrine system, causing infertility. The side effects of chemotherapy can be so terrible that they make patients feel that they no long own their own bodies; as the treatment proceeds, their bodies come to feel increasingly alien and troublesome. Ted Rosenthal underwent chemotherapy for his leukemia when that form of treatment was first introduced and the drugs used were less effective than those employed today. The side effects, though, are still as bad as they were then; nor has there been a change in the feelings of disconnection and despair—to the point of making the patient want to give up and die—that Rosenthal describes in the following poem:

Open one eye.
Suck thermometer; extend pulse; exchange water
    pitchers.

Feel skull for night hair-loss. Verify it in mirror.
Swallow thioguanine; eat breakfast; reread night
    poem
written in anger.
Consult physician; change pajamas; feed the fish.
    Water the chrysanthemums; straighten the
    picture; raise the dead.
Vomit the mind.
My dreams are beyond control!
Take a piss standing up; real; enter trio of doctors;
Any problems of any sort?
Not a one; finish piss.
My darling, for God's sake I give up.
How do I make you vanish?
Answer the phone; open other eye. Suck
    thermometer.
                         —Rosenthal (1973, p. 23)

Cancer patients fear chemotherapy more than any other treatment modality. Senator Hubert Humphrey called it "bottled death" (Howe, 1981, p. 30). The Israeli poet Abba Kovner, who wrote the following poem when he was hospitalized for a metastasized neck tumor, compares the colorless chemicals that drip into his body to death itself:

Transparence

Drip
Drip
Drips from above into his veins
Atropine colorless
Like death. Like the spelling of his name
In a foreign tongue

Dripping into any telephone receiver
To get an American answer caressing
An alien heart . . . .
                    —Kovner (1988a, p. 3, translated from
                    Hebrew by Barbara and Benjamin
                    Harshav).

The chemotherapeutic agents that are injected or put into an infusion are highly toxic and therapeutically effective only in carefully calibrated dosages. If too much medication is injected or if it is injected in the wrong place, the result can range from a painful inflammation of the veins, at a minimum, to a real life threat at worst. The side effects are often fearsome, even though each patient reacts differently to different chemotherapeutic agents.

Stoudemire (1983), himself a doctor with cancer, writes:

> Few physicians have any conception of the traumatic impact of a severely toxic regimen of chemotherapy. There is no way to describe the pain, fear, horror, and dread that the chemotherapy treatments evoked. The effects were physically and emotionally devastating. I suffered from gastritis and myalgias. I did not eat solid food for 4 or 5 days at a time. The tips of my fingers and soles of my feet became numb. I partially lost my sense of taste. . . .
>
> The associated nausea and vomiting were intractable at times. The first day of the cycle was the most severe. I would vomit and retch at 5-minute intervals for almost 8 hours. Eventually the vomiting would decrease to every 10 or 15 minutes. Often, I would have simultaneous diarrhea and abdominal cramping. I often fainted from fatigue, exhaustion and dehydration. Throughout these hospitalizations, nurses would usually close the door, "check in" every few hours and in general withdraw from my presence. Their inability to control the vomiting apparently made them feel helpless and inadequate. The chemotherapy treatments continued for five days every 3 weeks for 10 months and were then terminated.
>
> Every cycle of chemotherapy became a ritual of death and resurrection. No one could dread death itself more than I came to dread getting that medicinal "poison." There seemed to be absolutely nothing to look forward to except the day when I would get the final dose and complete the protocol. When I finally finished a cycle, the following day I would experience life with incredible emotional intensity. I would feel an almost euphoric exhilaration in having survived the ordeal and joy in just being alive; sights, sounds, colors were enhanced and incredibly vivid. The euphoria tended not to last long; I would soon start dreading the next "round" and sink back into my chronically morbid state of fear and depression [p. 382].

Herbert Howe (1981), a Harvard graduate student with a rare form of fibrosarcoma, describes how chemotherapy affected his identity:

> Over the last few weeks I pondered how chemo was ruining my life. By late fall I no longer considered myself a Harvard

graduate student researching and teaching international affairs. I was a cancer patient, totally dependent upon forces which I could neither understand nor influence. . . . "It's not that life is so unfair," I concluded, "but that it's so uncontrollable" [p. 105].

Vomiting and nausea are very common reactions to chemotherapy. During the course of treatment, however, the reflex to vomit may begin to appear even before the patient reenters the hospital or when he first sees the attending nurse. This anticipatory vomiting can be considered a disturbance of perception, with the patient anticipating the visceral response, initially stimulated by the aggressive treatment, and reacting to its perceptual triggers in the environment. This kind of anticipatory vomiting can still be active years after the treatment has been completed, especially when the patient must return to the hospital for regular medical examinations. Even though anticipatory vomiting constitutes a strong reaction against treatment, it is usually not so strong that treatment must be interrupted. Pharmacological management, active and passive relaxation techniques, hypnosis, and visualization techniques can successfully counteract anticipatory vomiting (Redd, 1989). Most patients who receive chemotherapy subsequently state that they would go through it again, and, in retrospect, they tend to develop a more positive view of it. When first confronted with chemotherapy, however, patients typically tend to feel that their essential vitality is being damaged through the treatment.

For some patients, marijuana can be used instead of an antiemetic drug to counteract nausea and vomiting. For Ted Rosenthal (1973), this obviously was an excellent idea:

Asparaginase, the drug that I have been on for the last couple of weeks, causes acute nausea that no drug, no pill will do anything to help. So my doctor came rushing in one day when I was lying on my back underneath this bottle of asparaginase and said "Do you have any weed? Do you have any access to weed?" And I said "What kind of weed do you mean?" and he said, "Grass, pot, marijuana." So I got some that night and I sat there and I decided to wait until I thought I was at my worst. I sat there with a bowl in my lap, ready to vomit, and a pipe of pot in my other hand. And just as I was about to let loose, I took a puff and, whee, it was gone. I felt fine. I went right in after two or three puffs and I ate a dozen crabs and a huge lobster and a piece of chocolate cake on top of that, then I went rushing back to the doctor the next day and told him and he said "Fantastic." So he has me on pot now [p. 59].

Since chemotherapeutic agents also attack healthy cells and especially the immune system, and since the discomfort of the side effects is
often initially much worse than the disease, the patient necessarily views
the treatment with ambivalence.

Both chemotherapy and radiation therapy have a profound effect on
food tolerance and thus on nutrition both during and often long after the
termination of the treatment. Monitoring the patient's weight can serve
either as reassurance that the disease is not yet out of hand or as a
dreaded affirmation that the disease is finally preparing to devour its
victim, a fantasy stemming from the metaphors associated with cancer
and made concrete by the wasting away of the terminal patient.

Chemotherapy, like radiotherapy, can be experienced by the patient
as devouring as the cancer itself. For, like radiotherapy, chemotherapy
destroys healthy cells as well as the diseased cancer cells. The feelings
that the threat of these powerful toxic chemicals evoke in patients will
determine the patients' responses and color their participation in the
treatment. The physical response to the medication is as to something
indigestible; and vomiting, the body's instinctive response to bad food, is
a common side effect. The oncologist who "feeds" the patient these toxins
is perceived, on one hand, as the sustainer of life but, on the other, as the
provider of "poisonous food." Yet, the patient remains strongly dependent
on the oncologist, whose knowledge can shorten or prolong life, and this
dependence makes it impossible for the patient to discharge aggression
toward the physician directly. The repression of aggression can become
psychologically toxic, just as the medicine is physiologically toxic. The
body retains the power to discharge toxicity by spitting it out, but the mind
has no such ability (Goldberg, 1981). The build-up of psychological toxicity
may, in time, make the relationship to the doctor/"food giver" as toxic to
the patient as the chemotherapy itself (Goldberg, 1981). The patient may
become silent, fearing that his anger is as perceptible as the reeking breath
caused by the treatment. In this situation, the doctor must actively reach
out to the patient to keep supportive communication going.

The patient's attempt to cure his nausea with a particular diet during
cancer therapy means that he has moved from his initially helpless
position, similar to that of an infant, to an understanding of his own active
role in treatment; this is a constructive move toward health. The patient
may learn to eat in a new way, for example, by eliminating processed
foods containing chemical additives and preservatives, or by finding a new
diet, or by changing his eating patterns. The patient thus learns to regulate
his food intake independent of his relationship to the provider of the "food
medicine," the doctor.

The 24-year-old patient John Baker, a successful long distance runner
described in the book *A Shining Season*, by William Buchanan (1978),

provides an apt example. During chemotherapy administered to fight his metastasized cancer of the testicles, Baker consistently vomited all his food. Afraid that he would lose so much weight and strength that we would be unable to meet the task he had set for himself in the little time left before his death, Baker discovered that if he prepared two sandwiches ahead of time he could beat the vomiting. He would vomit the first sandwich and then he would immediately eat the second one, which he then kept down. He could thereby control his food intake, keep his weight stable, and proceed with his task as a trainer for the school children he loved.

Another example is to be found in the book by the physician Anthony Sattilaro (1982), *Recalled by Life*. The author tells us how he battled his terminal cancer not only with traditional medical treatment, but also with a macrobiotic diet composed of brown rice, whole grains, beans, fresh vegetables, and fish, eaten at a commune where a positive, spiritual approach to life was pervasive. Several months into this regime, the course of Sattilaro's cancer halted and his body started to mend. Eventually he stopped the traditional medical treatment but continued with his chosen diet. Regular medical checkups have documented that five years later he had no sign of cancer left. Sattilaro took his physical well-being in his own hands, as he was accustomed to do as a doctor. The diet provided him not only with a physical cure, but also fostered a new feeling of wholeness and spiritual fulfillment, which had been missing from his life:

Macrobiotics had become my reason for hope; it was the thread from which my life hung, and though I often thought that it was no more reason for hope than was the remote chance of a miracle, I was now beginning to believe that a miracle was on its way. . . .

It had been just twelve months before that I was told that I had a terminal illness. I believed then that I would be dead before my fiftieth birthday. What followed that diagnosis was a series of tragedies: three operations, the loss of my testicles, the death of my father, the slow dismantling of my mother, and the long and bitter wait for my own imminent death. . . .

Soon Michio finished examining me and stood back. He looked at me in the way one does when one wants to remember someone's face.

"You don't have cancer anymore, Tony. You've beaten your disease," Michio said. With that he stood back and smiled.

Suddenly a wall of tension, desperation, pain and disappointment collapsed; joy rushed through me like healing waters. Everyone in the room was patting me on the back and congratulating me. I had done the impossible! I had licked a disease that was unbeatable by every measure I had believed in [pp. 137–140].

Howe (1981), the Harvard student, describes how his humor helped him to deal with the passivity forced upon him by the chemotherapy treatment:

> Immediately after Loring [chemotherapy nurse] left, I ran toward the bathroom. I started vomiting as I entered. Two hours later I limped back to bed.
>
> On Wednesday morning I finally did what I had often thought of doing during the last six months. During several chemo sessions . . . my breakfast nurse had appeared visibly nervous whenever I was around.
>
> I awoke with the sun. Soon the breakfast carts began clanking down the hallway. Still tasting the remains of nausea, I nevertheless grinned as I stumbled towards the closet. I pulled out my Ape-Face [mask].
>
> Back in bed, I slipped the rubberband attachment over my head and then pulled the blue blanket over my head . . . I could feel her getting closer and closer. Finally the magic moment as she pulled my blanket away.
>
> "Oh, shit. Oh, my God. Oh, no," she yelled and ran from the room. I smiled and lay back in bed. I had scored another victory against passivity and dependence [pp. 147–148].

Howe describes how he threw himself into running, boxing, weight lifting, and canoeing as a way of overcoming his sense of physical debilitation and psychological passivity.

Hair loss is one of the most threatening side effects of chemotherapy. Hair, the symbol of beauty, sensuousness, and fertility in a woman, and of strength and virility in a man, represents health and life. Losing one's hair, the most obvious change in the body, signals for most patients the loss of physical vitality and the beginning of the dying process. To be confronted with one's skull in the mirror is to see one's dying self. Even though the healthy hair cells recover soon after chemotherapy is concluded and the hair starts growing again, patients of all ages experience hair loss as a major threat. Shirley Sikes (1988) writes:

> When I took all the drugs, my hair fell out. I awoke one day and tried to comb it. As I moved the comb through my hair, huge chunks fell out. The comb became clogged. Hairs fell

over my face and settled on my lips as though they were
leaves falling from a tree.

My head looked like the top of the great, bald mountain. My
head looked like the plucked dome of that abandoned doll.

My head looked like a skull....

When my hair fell out, I bought a wig. I was terrified the wig
would fall off. People complimented me on my hair. At night,
when I took the wig off, my head was cold. I covered my
baldness with a scarf. I looked like a robot [p. 82].

Dora Hauri (1982), who had breast cancer, wanted to die:

November 7th 1979
Hairs, many hairs on my pillow. No, I don't want to play in
this tragedy. The doctors are like goblins playing a nasty game
with me. They poison and betray me. They talk me into the
idea that life without hair is still worth living. They get
satisfaction from prolonging my dying and try to make me
believe that they really want to help me. Without medication
my life would end soon. That's fine. I am afraid that I will not
make a self-death. I will let myself be talked out of it [p. 47].

Fiore (1979), himself a cancer survivor and a medical psychologist,
suggests carefully informing the patient of the positive effects of chemotherapy and the temporary nature of the hair loss before embarking on the
treatment:

They can say, "You will be receiving some very powerful
medicine capable of killing rapidly producing cells. Cancer is
the most rapidly producing cell, but there are other rapidly
producing cells such as hair. And since the medication cannot
tell the difference between hair and cancer cells, you may lose
some hair temporarily. Fortunately, your normal, healthy cells
can recover from the medication and reproduce themselves,
but the weak, poorly formed cancer cells cannot" [pp.
286–287].

Another feared concomitant of chemotherapy is being constantly
poked in the veins for blood or transfusions. The approach of the
technician makes Sikes (1988) want to hide, and she feels as if she were
reverting to childhood:

Finding a new vein was the hard thing. After so many weeks, and with only one arm (you shouldn't put needles in the arm where the nodes are gone) you find fresh veins are extremely dear. If the technician is not good with the butterfly (the smallest needle they can find), it is going to be tough. Poking and probing and no blood is what will happen.

You find yourself reverting to childhood. You want to run and hide when you see the wrong technician is coming to take your blood.

They don't want to see you either. "I hope it's not _____," they say, naming you. "It's too hard to get blood out of her."

In a way, I'm pleased. I've been singled out somehow [p. 84].

Although blood transfusions can become a necessity during any kind of cancer treatment or as a result of bleeding, they too can provoke the patient's fears and fantasies. In her poem "Dracula," Webster expresses her strong revulsion at the "stranger's blood" being pumped into her body: her fantasy is that, as with Dracula's victims, she is becoming a vampire:

Dracula

There is a part in Dracula
I'd like to sink my teeth in—
Lovely lady in lace,
terror and compliance,
tormented sexuality.
I succumb to his lust,
in turn lure men
to their destruction.
But this transfusion comes
like processed pig
liver, cased in plastic.
A sluggish start.
My vein resents
a stranger's blood.
A saline flush,
and I can watch
port wine drops
splash into dark magenta,
trail down
into my hand.
I can't look
this liver

in the eye.
My vein demands
more personal
connection.

—Webster (1980, p. 43)

The various cancer treatments affect the patient both internally and externally. The hair loss and loss of weight due to chemotherapy, the loss of limbs through surgery, and the overall debilitating effects of both the disease and the treatments can produce radical physical changes. These make cancer patients feel estranged from themselves and strangers to familiar friends.

Gitanjali, a 16-year-old Indian girl with terminal cancer, secretly wrote many poems expressing her hurt, fears, longings, and wishes. She hid those poems from her parents, fearing that her mother would be much too hurt if she knew that her daughter was fully aware of her fate. These poems, which were found after her death, were the only way for the young patient to express the strong emotions she could not share with anybody.

In "The Naked Shock," she relates her first appearance back in high school after having undergone intense cancer treatment in the hospital:

The Naked Shock

Gitanjali has come
Gitanjali has come
Is the general roar
In the School Corridor
From one friend to another
And to those
She still matters most
Gitanjali!!!
Is she Gitanjali ? ?
They stare with a naked shock
But they say not much
For the fear of hurting
Whom they still love as much.

Gitanjali is not unaware
Of her beauty shorn
But swallows the pain
With her pride
And offers her smile

> After all ...
> Illness too is
> A gift from God
> And Gitanjali accepts it
> With grace and in good stride.
> —Gitanjali (in Badruddin, 1982, p. 27)

If therapy is successful, the patient should come into a remission. It can be a partial or a full remission. On one hand, remission is a new lease on life for the cancer patient, as Alsop (1973) writes:

> "Remission of sins"—the phrase tantalized my memory for several days. The phrase was suggested, of course, by the "remission," alas temporary, which with luck followed a session of chemotherapy. I couldn't remember the rest of it or where it came from. Finally, Tish supplied the rest: "remission of sins, resurrection of the dead, and life everlasting." From the Credo, of course [p. 53].

On the other hand, that it is temporary fills Alsop with dread:

> It had always rather irritated me, when John Glick told me that if I went into remission after a course of chemotherapy I could lead a "normal life." Normal—shmormal, I told him. To live from blood test to blood test, from marrow test to marrow test, always knowing that the day would come when the tests would spell "death"—what kind of normal life was that? [p. 123].

If treatment—surgery, radiation therapy, or chemotherapy—is offered in the first treatment phase, then its goal is to cure or arrest the disease. This goal generally generates optimism in spite of the bad side effects of treatment and allows a certain degree of freedom in the communication of the doctor to patient. In this situation, the patient's anxiety can be lessened if the doctor answers his questions and adequately informs him of everything he can expect to undergo in the course of his therapy. In this phase, talks between doctor and patient generally focus on the successful treatment of similar tumors in other patients. The doctor, however, should be on guard not to tell the patient more than he wants to know. Today's patient realizes that the only way to really measure the success of a cancer treatment is observation of the course of the illness. Thus, when a new form of treatment is initiated in the second treatment phase, the patient knows that the cancer has progressed after the first round of treatment and that more powerful agents are being used to attack the disease. In this case, communication between doctor and patient can become difficult, as we shall see in the next chapter.

5

FEARS IN THE
FACE OF CANCER
AND ITS TREATMENT

They train you at the hospital not to think in terms of the future at all. They never speak in terms of dates or lengths of time and they don't promise you anything. Therefore when they give you good news, all they are essentially telling you is that you're not dead. All those people who say that you are predictable and that you will die in the same way that everyone else dies, they are right. I resented that at first. I resented them saying "Oh you are at the two week stage. You're feeling, doing this. You're free. You're at the angry stage. I understand that. You're depressed. You're lost. Three and one half weeks after you find this out you always feel lost" [Rosenthal, 1973, p. 24].

Patients who have to undergo intensive treatment for cancer often experience the treatment as a massive assault on the integrity and coherence of the self. This assault may entail various consequences. The most prominent is the loss of a sound feeling of self-confidence and self-respect, which may become so severe as to lead to feelings of being psychologically extinguished, to panic attacks and, in rare cases, to psychotic episodes. To reestablish equilibrium in the menaced self, patients sometimes mobilize primitive defense mechanisms that may themselves create considerable difficulties (Meerwein, 1987a).

For the tumor patient, fears signal a dreaded loss of outer and inner integrity, both bodily and psychic, and usher in the mobilization of the psychological functions that are needed to reestablish this integrity. The fears derive from various sources. They are a mixture of residual neurotic fears, reality-based fears, and fears of death. They include most of the fantasies related to the person's particular "cancer" metaphor, such as fears of being abandoned, of social isolation, of persecution, of being overtaken by one's own inner badness, of passive surrender, or of being overpowered by uncontrollable forces. Then there are fears of sustaining narcissistic damage, of being sickened by radiation and chemotherapy or mutilated by surgery, and thus of being left only with envy for the healthy. There are the realistic fears of losing one's autonomy and one's ability to enjoy life, of pain, and of having a relapse and progressing into incurability. Then there are the terrifying fears—of death, of psychic and physical annihilation. To these can be added the fear of losing control over reality or of becoming shunned by significant others because of psychophysical disintegration and the revulsion it may provoke.

Patients do not, however, stand helpless before these fears. They have a variety of ways of dealing with them. Denial, rationalization, avoidance, repression, and reaction formation are the most common psychological defenses that cancer patients use to protect and reconstitute the integrity of the self (Meerwein, 1986). These defense mechanisms, however, are rarely good enough to keep the patient's fears under control. Usually some of the fear persists despite the patient's defenses and takes the form of free floating anxiety. It is the task of the doctor and the psychologist to recognize these fears and to help the patient control them. Patients today expect their treatment plans to include a fight against their anxiety. They realize that only a more or less fear-free personality is sufficiently strong to fight and win the war against cancer. Unfortunately, more patients than doctors believe in this holistic approach to medicine.

The most powerful weapons with which to fight the cancer patient's fear are anticipatory discussion of possible sources of fear, openness, explanations, object constancy (meaning that the doctor stays emotionally and physically available), truthfulness, and enlisting the patient's active participation in the rehabilitation process from the earliest stage. The prescription of anxiolytica (antianxiety agents) is, in some difficult cases, also necessary.

DENIAL

If denial is still strongly operative after the initial denial that usually follows the patient's hearing the diagnosis, that is, if it persists during the later phases of treatment, increases with the progression of the illness, or reappears in the terminal phase, then it must be recognized as the outcome of poor medical guidance (Meerwein, 1985a). In this maladaptive denial, the patient consciously splits off all feelings connected to fear and suffering. This denial requires psychological help and should not be supported by the doctor or treatment team as it so often is. Further, if the patient becomes the victim of a maladaptive denial originally suggested by the doctor, then their relationship will be seriously undermined and the patient's feeling of self-worth will be badly injured. Deprived of an honest relationship, the patient begins to hate the doctor, who may have to withdraw from the treatment.

Like every human being, the cancer patient is part of a web of human relationships that include family members, doctors, nurses, friends, and other patients. In this circle of relationships, denial invariably has an important social function. Patients who deny do so to protect not only the self but also their relationships as well. The denial has the function of establishing a picture of the patient as a frank, fear-free, cooperative human being, who does not bother the doctor and others with discomforting questions. It is meant to secure the badly needed support of those closest to the patient by keeping the people around him in good spirits and thereby preventing their withdrawal. The forces behind this socially determined denial remains unconscious in the patient most of the time, Rollin's (1976) perceptions quoted in the previous chapter notwithstanding. It is, therefore, very important that the doctor recognize it so that it does not obstruct the patient–doctor dialogue. If a collusion occurs between doctor and the patient to keep the denial going, the patient may inwardly start to develop intense fears as well as feelings of isolation and depression.

DEPRESSION FOLLOWING THE RELINQUISHMENT OF DENIAL

Depression always accompanies cancer. Its appearance signals that the defense of denial can no longer protect the self, and the patient must admit, "I can deny it no longer, I am suffering from cancer." Depression is a necessary phase of the working-through process in an illness like cancer. If feelings of isolation and fear of the loss of supportive relationships are connected to the depression, we call it an anaclitic depression (Spitz, 1965). If the depression is associated with the loss of the good feeling of self, of security, and of ego strength and brings with it the further loss of both the active and passive capacity for love, then we call it a reactive depression (Bibring, 1961). In the cancer patient we usually find a mixture of these two types of depressions (Meerwein, 1984).

Depression should be distinguished from the mourning reaction in which patients withdraw into themselves in order to deal with their loss

(Freud, 1917). People who mourn have fewer feelings of guilt and shame than do depressed people. They may be able to express their mourning in tears, they are never totally hopeless, and they often retain their sense of humor.

Most often their cancer patients are ashamed of his depression. That is why they denies it to the people around them or even represses their own awareness of it, in which case the depression changes from a manifest to a latent one. Latently depressed patients are "easy," quiet patients; thus, the problem is often overlooked. Overlooking it, in turn, intensifies these patients' bad feelings about themselves and adds to their emotional suffering. When patients are depressed, communication is especially important; and the doctor should make every effort to reach them. Some doctors believe that they can "trick" the depression through selective or total denial and need not treat it. More often than not, the contrary is true. The physician's denial of the depression only makes it worse, for it fosters ever deeper feelings of isolation in the patients. If patients can talk openly with their doctors, their depression may be alleviated.

Often, on hearing the diagnosis of cancer or on beginning intensive treatment, patients feel, instead of depression, a sudden emptiness, frequently attended by great anxiety and hopelessness. Patients feel that their very being is so threatened that they no longer have control over the mysterious, terrifying happenings that originate both within them and in the external world (Meerwein, 1987a).

Diggelmann (1979) describes this sudden emptying:

> December 30th, 1978
> How do you feel? As if I have to feel something. There is only one answer. I don't feel anything. I don't feel sick. I don't feel afraid. I don't feel the future. Whatever feelings exist are growing like flowers under the snow. If somebody asks me, "Didn't you feel anything positive since November 23rd, when you learned that your life is limited?" then I will have to answer: I always knew it was limited. But is it really limited? Or is it maybe, after all, unlimited? If I at least feel sick, someone asks. Maybe that's the illness, not to feel sick. The only honest answer is, no, I don't feel sick. I don't feel myself at all. Death comes earlier, or later [pp. 23–24].

Somewhat later in his illness, Diggelmann emphasizes the loneliness and hopelessness that follow upon the emptying:

> The last days have been marked by deep fears and hidden depression and tears. I have never been as lonely as in the last

few days. It is a long time since I have had such a basic fear, that I would never be able to go home again [p. 104].

The continuation of the malignant process that necessitates the second treatment phase often fosters depressive reactions in the patient. Alsop (1973) describes these as follows:

> Between spurts of reading, I would doze, and read my mail, and read some more, and doze again. Except for Tish and Nicky and little Andrew [wife and sons], I wanted to see no one. It was not so much that I was depressed; I don't remember being particularly sad, though of course I now thought I was quite likely to die quite soon. I was just indifferent. I didn't much care about anything.
>
> It wasn't that I felt desperately ill physically, or even desperately depressed. I felt, instead, a kind of weariness, a vast indifference. In my head during this time there was a sort of continual background music—or rather, background ca- cophony—not exactly a headache but a kind of murmuring unpleasantness. And a very bad thing happened: I could hardly read at all. After half an hour, the page would blur, and the cacophony in my head would mount from a murmur to a shout [p. 121].

The depressive reaction, with its attendant muting of emotional responses, can go so far that even the threat of death fails to evoke an emotional reaction:

> I was pretty sure by this time that my cause was hopeless too, but it didn't bother me half as much as it had during my first stay at NIH, when I still enjoyed those picnics in the waiting room, and drinking martinis, and reading, and laughing, and seeing my friends. The second time I was in NIH, I enjoyed nothing. I did not want to die, but I didn't want desperately *not* to die [p. 133].

The East German writer Brigitte Reimann (1984) describes the symptoms of her depression without realizing what they are:

> September 21th, 1971
> I don't know what happened to me, nor does my psychia- trist, who patiently takes me apart, seem to understand it—in any case for the past several months I have been living in a

strange semi-consciousness. I can't write any longer; I can't read, can't understand what I read; I don't dare to go outside, to talk to people, a panic fear of being alone, the feeling that I am moving in an abstract world.

December 29th, 1971
   My lady hasn't done anything for months, that means: the author hasn't done anything for months. That's how long this devilish semi-consciousness has lasted, and now I even know why: a dark presentiment has come true now. Cancer, which can no longer be operated on; I should have been dead by now for at least a half a year. But look, I am still alive and I hope to make it for some more years with the help of herb brandy and trust in God. This is just between us. In any event I want to, must and can work again [p. 344].

Reimann's depression is associated with her strong denial of her cancer. At every stage of the illness, she is surprised by the deterioration in her condition. Her depressive symptoms disappear when her straight-talking doctor reclarifies her medical status.

   The course of Reimann's depression suggests the complexities of depression in the cancer patient. Depression is usually the first response following the relinquishment of the initial adaptive denial. As long as the patient denied his illness at that stage, he had no cause to feel depressed. As the cancer progresses, however, and its debilitating symptoms and intrusive treatment make full denial impossible, any denial that remains will persistently affect both the patient's inner perception and his resonance with external reality. A sense of dissonance, of living a lie, is created. It cuts the patient off from his deepest feelings and from those around him who do not share his pretense. It fosters alienation, loneliness, and depression. The only remedy is a return to reality, however painful. While recognition of the illness will obviously not alleviate the cancer patient's fears, it will bring a modicum of relief.

   Nonetheless, depression is a constant in cancer. As the account by Mullan (1983), the physician who saw the x-ray of his lung cancer, shows, depression can crop up at any point in the disease and be brought on by almost any of the various aspects of the illness and its treatments. Mullan describes how his depression repeatedly resurfaced during a long hospital stay during which he underwent numerous surgical interventions and other treatments:

   In the weeks that followed I was to weep frequently and suddenly without immediate cause. The disease and its treatment so stripped me of my defenses that any event with the least bit of emotional content caused me to cry. I cried over some television news stories (Vietnam was falling at the time) as well as over many kind letters that I received from friends. Talking with Judy about our future was always interrupted by a tearful episode or two on my part. While the tears were honest and cathartic they were also an annoying impediment to almost any serious conversation. In retrospect I suppose they were tears of impotence and anger, tears of a spirit that had been blind-sided by disease. As the weeks passed, my raw emotions became rawer and my sense of self-pity deepened [p. 37].

I only know that during this time I felt blighted physically and overrun psychologically. I am sure that deep within me I was furious at the fates which had brought me to my knees in youth. Had I had the energy and a target, or even a surrogate target, I imagine I would have broken out in rage. But I was past being angry. What I do remember feeling was despair. My glass, it seemed to me now, was indeed half empty [p. 42].

Yet while being in the hospital made Mullan feel depressed, being released did not alleviate his depression. On the contrary, the prospect of leaving the protective environment for an unknown situation and a new role in a new home intensified his depression to the point of his fantasizing suicide:

Friends in the hospital congratulated me on my impending departure. I had made it through therapy and, after two months, was going home, where things would be better. I didn't feel that way about it at all. I had arrived at the hospital seemingly healthy, mentally intact, and ready to do battle. Now I was leaving the hospital in a wheelchair, emaciated, unable to swallow, troubled by breathing, and acutely depressed. I didn't miss my trips to the chemotherapy unit, but my last morning of radiation therapy, the day before I was to leave the hospital, I suffered an incredible spasm of anxiety. Crying did no good. Vomiting, spitting, and belching were in no way cathartic. There seemed to be no avenue of escape from the constant fear and nausea that I felt.

I began studying the screens on the two windows in my private ninth-floor room. Would I have the strength to remove them? Was there anything that I could lift that was heavy enough to punch through them? I didn't care so much where I landed or who discovered that I was missing as I did what the mechanism would be to get the windows cleared. I still had enough sense of what was going on inside my head to call the nursing station and ask for help. It was seven in the morning. Judy would be busy with Meghan, so I called Dad and asked him to come to the hospital as soon as he could. He was there by eight o'clock. In the meantime, a corpsman named Al who had been a steady friend sat beside my bed and held my hand. I hugged Dad when he arrived.

I had no idea of what was happening that day except that my life, or what was left of it, was coming to a head. In spite of my abhorrence of the hospital I feared leaving it. The burning radiation and the noxious chemicals were what I had come to believe in—in spite of their poisonous effects. Deep within me I could not accept being cut adrift to fend for myself. I had become a slave of my therapies. Even though I understood the need to terminate them, I think I would have doggedly climbed onto the radiation table daily until the rays had burned a hole clean through me. Leaving Tower Nine through the window became more appealing than abandoning the poisons. I wanted to live at any cost, so badly, in fact, that I was prepared to die [pp. 57–58].

Though depression cannot be eliminated in cancer, it can be alleviated. Noll (1984), who became more and more depressed as his symptoms became more severe, tells in his diary how he coped with his bad mood by planning a visit to his close friend Max Frisch, and by thinking of his two daughters, for whom he had warm and protective feelings:

July 25, 1982

Everything is difficult now, even my breathing. My inability to make decisions is at its height. I don't leave the house even though it is not raining. Nothing stimulates or tempts me. My dictation, the illness, the pain, my thoughts about death, everything has become routine. . . . Tomorrow I will visit Max Frisch in Bergona. From the lowest point movement can only go up. This last span of time is asking more than every earlier one. What will happen with my profession, my illness and my dying. And to those who will not have me any more, mostly to Rebekka and Sibylle [grown daughters]. I constantly think of these two. Somehow I would like to leave them a safe world, which is not possible. Constantly I keep thinking of new pet names to add to the old ones [p. 246].

Noll's account is instructive to the cancer physician and treatment team. It illustrates what can be done to alleviate a patient's depression despite the ravages of the disease, the long suffering, and the overriding fear of death. The empathy and caring that are needed can and should be provided by the physician and treatment team as well as by family and friends.

AGGRESSION AND PROJECTION

As is amply documented in many of the foregoing quotations, aggression also accompanies cancer. Aggression can be manifested either introjectively or projectively. Patients who work it through introjectively feel that they are bad, and a depressive state may ensue. For patients who work it through projectively, the environment becomes bad and hostile, and they feel attacked, devalued, or even destroyed. Patients who are able to express negative emotions like anger, hate, and aggression, or to show frustration and feelings of disappointment, might, according to some authors, have a better chance at survival than patients who can show only positive feelings (Baltrusch, 1969).

The rage of cancer patients derives from the threat that the disease poses to the integrity of the self. Diggelmann (1979) clearly identifies a common feeling among cancer patients—the hatred of being controlled by others: "With tears I flushed my fear out of my body, as well as my hatred for everyone who has control over me. I don't want to deny that it was hate" (p. 60).

The issue of control is important for all patients, but most especially for adolescents. Too often, appointments are made, and treatments scheduled, with unnecessary brusqueness, as though the timetable were dictated down to the minute by the logic of the best medical wisdom. With adolescent patients, greater compliance can be gained by giving them some leeway in scheduling and other nonessential aspects. It is important to ask all patients for their own suggestions about how and when treatment may be best delivered.

As the illness progresses, subtle and not so subtle struggles over control become more pronounced as the patient faces an ever-increasing loss of control over various portions of his life. What begins as perhaps no more than a series of interruptions in life threatens to turn into a state of permanent invalidism, in which one's say over one's activities is ever more severely curtailed. Late in the illness the patient may even be faced with the loss of control over his bodily functions and ultimately with the loss of control over his ego. The resulting conflicts often are played out with the medication, for this is the one area of life over which the patient still retains some control.

Thus, whether, or how, to take what kind of medicine often becomes the battleground for long pent-up frustrations over the progressive loss of control inherent in the illness. These battles are frequently fought not only with medical staff but also with the family.

But it is not only over the medication that the patient finally expresses anger. Almost any aspect of cancer can evoke anger. Diggelmann (1979) describes the unanswerable questions that made him angry and fostered feelings of depression:

> What remains are daily questions, such as: when can I leave the hospital to go back to my apartment which I furnished with lots of love and which I soon will no longer recognize? How can I go on living with my story? I will need to change in a lot of ways. As I said, I can no longer bear the questions about my health. I could even become rude and say: Save me your stupidity! If you don't know, then there is no need to ask, and if you do know, then please don't ask [pp. 94–95].

Some cancer patients lash out at any available target. Mostly these aggressive outbursts are directed at persons who do not respond to the needs of the patient's self for sensitive understanding and empathy. The patient's expectations are thus disappointed, and his fragile sense of self-worth is again badly injured; the ensuing outburst is an expression of pent-up narcissistic rage.

Feelings of aggression can be experienced as a burden in the doctor-patient relationship, especially if the aggression stems from envy that the patient feels toward his healthy doctor. These feelings can become especially intense if patient and doctor are of the same generation and the patient's illness is progressive.

Although not all cancer patients express aggression, narcissistic rage, envy, or feelings of distrust, these feelings and the projections they engender are feared by the treatment team no less than by the patient, since medical ethics prevent the doctor and the nurses from responding with counteraggression. All people in the patient's environment have to try not to take the aggression directed toward them personally, but to realize that it represents the injury to the patient's personality caused by the cancer. The aggression is a "scream for help," a reaction formation against feelings of helplessness.

Michie's (1980) vivid, imaginative description of her anger gives us a good sense of the strong, pervasive rage that many cancer patients feel. In the following passage she describes how "A.F." was born:

I decided that I would probably skip the first three phases and plunge headlong into a deep depression. The denial and anger and bargaining stages seemed too irrational for a cool-headed lady like me. Facts are facts, malignant cells are malignant. "Why me?" is so obviously answered by "Why *not* me?" Getting mad at God seemed so childish.

But anger came in a strange free floating form. There must be someone to blame, someone who robbed me of precious time—the very prime of my life. My anger, free floating, gradually took an animal form. A tiny albino falcon appeared over the door of my hospital room, a vicious fellow with pink eyes and long pink talons. I named him A.F., which stood for Albino Falcon and for Anger, Free Floating. He was ready to attack anyone who abused me in any way—callous nurses, bearers of inedible meals, inconsiderate visitors, or cleaning personnel who might wake me from a nap.

He rode on the back of my wheelchair or stretcher when I was transported for tests or examinations, looking for callousness or carelessness in any form. For four days no one was callous or careless. A.F. was getting frantic and larger. He began flapping wildly around the room. Clearly he would have to attack an innocent, if a proper villain could not be found soon.

Monday morning the nurse announced that at 1:30 that afternoon I had an appointment at radiation oncology where I would discuss a proposed course of radiation therapy. A.F. and I were jubilant—a perfect villain! A.F. and I settled down, he to sharpen his talons and I to ponder my hatred of radiation and all doctors and technicians who practiced it [p. 414].

Sometimes, as we see in Diggelmann's (1979) statements, anger and depression alternate or commingle in the cancer patient's psyche. Often, however, the conscious experience and open expression of anger will protect the patient from severe depression, as is suggested by the lively, self-amused tone of Michie's account of her pugnacious attitude.

FEAR OF ENVY

Cancer patients are afraid and ashamed of their envy. As we have seen, envy is most often directed toward healthy people, who have whole, intact bodies and who are free to come and go as they wish. Envy can become especially strong when the patient readily identifies with the healthy person (e.g., a doctor of the same age) and when he or she is dependent on that person. Often envy is directed toward a particularly close nurse, doctor, or family member. Diggelmann (1979) is well aware of his envy of his wife:

> I do B. [wife] wrong. B. thinks I hate her. . . . I am jealous, envious, nothing more. I would like to drive home with her; I would like to put a record on [p. 59].

Envy can also be directed toward a stranger who is, or seems to be, proud of the organ the patient has lost, as the following quote by Rollin (1976) shows:

> Months later, on a short holiday, at a pool in Key Biscayne, Florida, I was wearing my new prosthesis inside a specially sewn-in pocket in my bathing suit top (which was also stitched up an extra inch in the middle to hide the still puffy pink scar), so I no longer had the "prosthesis problem" to distract me. Time had gone by and it was a beautiful day and I lay on the deck chair with the sun high and hot overhead and my mind was far from the place on my chest where a breast had been. Then I looked up and saw a girl walk by in an extremely brief fuchsia bikini who began to strut, sort of, around the edge of the pool. She had very large breasts. I started to read, but every time I looked up I could see her sashaying back and forth toward the diving board and back and forth again. I tried to keep on reading, but she kept strutting and I kept looking up, and before I realized what had happened to me I was sobbing horribly. I had sunglasses, luckily, to hide my eyes, but no tissues, so I stumbled inside and ran up to the hotel room. It took about an hour before I was ready to leave the room, and I never did make it back to the pool.
>
> That incident was no worse than several similar stabs of breast envy that had happened early on. But it hit me harder because it occurred when I no longer expected to feel that way. As I began to feel less awful about what had happened, I think I unconsciously expected it to "end"—the way my friend Joanna's broken hip had ended. These incidents reminded me that, although I felt better about what had happened and would no doubt, grow to feel still better, "what had happened" would never really end. Not ever [pp. 179–180].

Both Diggelmann and Rollin were aware of their envy and discussed it and dealt with it. Most cancer patients are less aware of their negative emotions, for example, Maya, a 14-year-old girl, whom I saw while she was hospitalized for the treatment of her terminal acute leukemia. In an art therapy session, Maya drew a picture of a freaky-looking girl. She entitled it "Does Not Find a Man Anymore," which she associated with herself. Maya was angry with her 16-year-old sister for not visiting enough, and her envy focused on her sister's many boyfriends. On an unconscious level, Maya realized that chemotherapy would not cure her leukemia and that she would never be able to marry as her healthy sister would. Her envy of her beloved sister also lay behind the title of another picture, "A Murder," which depicts a bleeding person. Discussing her pictures in therapy relieved Maya of the shame and guilt she felt at having harbored these envious feelings, which she feared would destroy her previously close, loving relationship with her sister.

This poem, by the adolescent Indian girl Gitanjali, describes the feeling of envy very clearly:

The Window-Pane

Whenever I feel
weary or depressed
or I'm in pain.
I just sit by myself
and look out through
the window-pane.

The sky looks
unblemished,
just like my soul.
Yet at times, its
spotted with dark
clouds of envy that
float in me, for the
birds that soar.

Here, I lie, helplessly
tied to my bed,
awaiting ...
the death sentence!
neither caring nor daring
to welcome my guest.
                    —Gitanjali (in Badruddin, 1982, p. 90)

Gitanjali and Maya are in their adolescence. Debilitated by terminal cancer, they can no longer go from one place to the other, or fly away like the birds. At this age, when the need for the independent discovery of the world is at its height and sensuous feelings awaken, these adolescent patients must repress all desire in order to survive. They feel envious of their healthy peers. Drawing and writing offered these girls an opportunity to deal actively with their fears and hopes and provided them with a hold on life.

GUILT

The subjective definition and experience of the illness are, for most people who have cancer, especially important. Human beings have a need for causality, and they tend to connect the conflicts of life to the development of their illness (Meerwein, 1986a). Cancer patients often blame themselves for their illness. It is usually difficult for them to sustain such self-blame, but the need to make some sense of their illness will move them to raise the subject in psychotherapy sessions.

Self-blame is evident in Mullan's (1983) search for the reasons behind his cancer:

> Guilt, also, was a theme in the search for a reason for my cancer. My plummet from youth and health to the depths of cancer must have been caused by something I had done . . . what was it? What act of hubris had I been guilty of? What principle, what ethic had I offended by my behavior? What had I done wrong? I never found sense or solace in these thoughts but I did entertain them. I mention them only to suggest that for me, as perhaps for others, the search for blame is a natural and almost instinctive reaction to unforeseen disaster [pp. 42–43].

Lying in the hospital after her mastectomy, Maxi Wander (1980) also ponders whether her sins have not brought on her disease: "Sometimes I ask myself whether it had to happen because *He* wanted to punish me for my vanity. Just accept it now, *He* says, don't rebel against it any more!" (p. 72).

Patients with masochistic tendencies seek confirmation for their self-blame, whereas those with more hysterical character traits tend to deny or repress such thoughts. Both types of patients, however, are relieved to hear their doctor or therapist reflect their embarrassing thoughts, "I understand that you wonder why you have cancer. But today we know so little about this illness that we can't say for sure whether your ideas are right or not." Acceptance or rejection of his theories of the genesis of his cancer is less important to the patient than that the doctor or therapist take the question seriously and try to understand it in the here and now. As a matter of fact, if the doctor agrees with a psychogenetic interpretation, he supports the patient's guilt feelings: if he rejects these thoughts completely, the patient feels misunderstood and not taken seriously. Empathy is the most powerful tool for resolving the question of guilt.

Guilt feelings can also evolve out of the immediate circumstances of the illness. Patients may be jealous, and therefore angry, at the healthy members of their family, angry at the people who do not respect their emotional needs, or even angry at God, who let all this happen in spite of faith in Him. All these angry feelings provoke guilt. The deeply religious 16-year-old Gitanjali writes how her intense feelings of guilt undermine her faith:

The Moment of Truth

Gitanjali is dead
Gitanjali is dead
People are whispering around
A horror of shock
But the moment of truth
That's all
It's all about

Foolish are those
Who shed tears
Mingled with sorrow and pain
Little do they realize
The joy that is mine
Free of torture
Free of pain
And free of guilt
That shook my faith
                    —Gitanjali (in Badruddin, 1982, p. 35).

DEPENDENCY AND AUTONOMY

Cancer patients are very aware of the extent of their illness even if they do not always show it openly. The sicker they become, the stronger is the wish to depend on the protection of the doctor, the treatment team, and the family. This wish is a benign regression. The wish, however, is often an ambivalent once, connected to many fears. For example, the patient may fear that the more dependent he becomes, the less capable he will be of independent action, and thus the more easily he can be manipulated or ignored by the doctor and treatment team. If these fears are not recognized and if the patient feels left out of the decision-making process, dependency needs become painful.

The deeply regressed, passive, infantilized patient is often a convenient one for the staff to have. Such a patient, however, not only develops regressive fears, but also feelings of shame and anger. These feelings he usually turns against himself, thus becoming even more depressed. In an attempt not to disrupt the relationship with the doctor, the patient will often develop a malignant regression (Meerwein, 1985a). He then withdraws totally and passively lets the nursing care happen, without participation, nor active rejection. The more actively the patient can be included in his treatment, the less he tends to become depressed (Fiore, 1979).

Alsop (1973) compares his sudden dependency on his wife with his dependence on his nanny when he was a little boy:

> I was dependent above all on Tish [wife], and in a way that I had not been dependent on any human being since Aggie Guthrie took care of me when I was very sick as a little boy. I was dependent on Tish not only for edible tidbits, martinis, books, and the like, but for a sort of unspoken emotional sustenance—for the squeeze of a warm hand in a time of darkness and fear. In time, I got used to this sense of dependence, and I even came, in a way, for the first time in my life, to enjoy it. Tish, knowing me, knew that I resented being dependent, and the emotional sustenance she gave me was therefore always unspoken [p. 53].

Obviously such total dependence on the part of an adult, independent person fosters aggression, and the cancer patient's doctors and treatment team should be prepared for an aggressive reaction.

> At first my dependence on other people annoyed me. It more than annoyed me, it infuriated me. I hate being dependent and have fought against it all my life. Perhaps it is something in the genes [p. 54].

The strong dependency cancer patients develop on their physicians is described by Alsop:

> I was dependent—deeply dependent, and for my very life—
> on John Glick [his physician], and it was John, not I, who
> decided when I could have my I.V. removed (after ten days or
> so, an I.V. becomes a hateful encumbrance) or what treatment
> I should have, or whether I could go home and what I could do
> when I got there [p. 56].

Cancer patients also become strongly dependent on the entire protective environment of the hospital. The hospital becomes a containing environment similar in many ways to the mother–infant relationship. It frees patients of all responsibility and gives them the opportunity to regress for a limited time.

Lorde (1980) describes the protective environment of the hospital:

> I was very anxious to go home. But I found also, and couldn't
> admit at the time, that the very bland whiteness of the hospital
> which I railed against and hated so, was also a kind of
> protection, a welcome insulation within which I could continue
> to non-feel. It was an erotically blank environment within
> whose undifferentiated and undemanding and infantilizing
> walls I could continue to be emotionally vacant—psychic
> mush—without being required by myself or anyone to be
> anything else [p. 46].

The East German writer Reimann (1984) expresses a similar dependence on the hospital's containing environment:

> Since I've come back from the hospital I haven't been able
> to write a single line. I longed for the hospital, the white coats,
> the non-responsibility, the routine non-day with its non-
> demands; . . . for the "magic mountain" atmosphere of the
> hospital [p. 339].

Rollin (1978) describes her regressive self in the hospital environment:

> Now I was in the monster's stomach. And it wasn't so bad.
> He had a nice little bed there for me, with sides, like a crib, and
> plenty to eat. It was warm, and I was sleepy. "Betty was such
> a happy baby," my mother used to say. In the monster's
> stomach I was happy and good. I was also cute and I smiled
> and I cooed and obeyed and everyone loved me. And I wasn't
> afraid any more, because the thing I was afraid of had

happened. Now I could just lie there and let the grown-ups worry [p. 92].

Interestingly, most of the renditions of the hospital as a protective environment are written by women patients after a mastectomy. If the mastectomy patient can experience the hospital, with its empathic female nurses, as a soothing place where she is allowed to regress temporarily and need not immediately confront herself and her loss, then the mourning process for the lost breast can evolve slowly and organically. On the other hand, if the patient experiences the hospital environment as unempathetic and unprotective and feels alone and emotionally rejected or ignored, then her already damaged narcissistic self is further undermined, fostering a depressive reaction before the patient has sufficiently recovered from the operation's physical effects to cope with it. Lorde (1980) conveys the importance of the female support she received from her many loving friends:

> I woke up in the recovery room after the biopsy colder than I can remember ever having been in my life. I was hurting and horrified. . . .
> From the time I woke up to the slow growing warmth of Adrienne's and Bernice's and Deanna's and Michelle's and Frances's coats on the bed I felt Beth Israel Hospital wrapped in a web of woman love and strong wishes of faith and hope for the whole time I was there, and it made self-healing more possible, knowing I was not alone [pp. 27, 29].

Helen Webster's poem brings home the importance of the patient's need to be able to regress in the hospital and how distressing the intrusive and overefficient technical regimen of the modern hospital can be.

They Don't Want Me To Sleep

They don't want me
to sleep.
When I do,
they wake me,
drip another
bottle in my vein,
feed me a pill,
check my vital signs.
I'm very clever,
Sleep when they

least suspect.
They bring me lunch.
I say, "thank you,"
and sleep.
They ask me
to watch the bottle
drip. I promise,
and sleep.
Night and day
the loudspeaker
outside my room
broadcasts coded
messages.
I know they turn
it louder when
I begin to sleep.
Throughout the night
they examine me
to see
if I'm still alive.
So far, I surprise
them
                    —Webster (1980, p. 42).

The resulting depression can become malignant and be accompanied by thoughts of suicide and death. If this happens, professional help may be needed to enable the patient to regain self-confidence and face her loss.

6

PROGRESSION

OF THE

CANCER

Maya Beutler (1980), the Swiss writer with a neck tumor, writes:

"It [the tumor] came back," I said, and with my right hand I
point to my neck. . . .

How did he [husband] ask: "Who told you?" *Who?* I look
at him and feel that I am losing more and more of my
perspective, no, my control. Why is Pierre [husband] so
controlled? Did Fink [physician] tell him something, yes, I am
sure, yes, I am being deceived, they act as if I am not here. A
minor. "Did Fink call?" I ask. At the same time I feel like
locking myself in quickly, for ever, like slamming the bathroom
door shut and screaming, "The rest is my own personal
business, my own individual business, go on alone, leave, yes,
just disappear, I am too proud to live out the script you planned
for me. I will shape the tiny little bit of life I have left myself."

Pierre comes towards me, I suddenly understand that he
wants to hug me, I retreat a step: "Since when have you
known?" I ask neutrally, yes, that's how everything sounds.
Pierre suddenly holds his hand in front of his eyes: "Stop it," he
says, I hear him breathing quickly. *Holding back tears,* no he
would like to hold back time, "Nine days," nine days I was
deceived. I stand still and cross my arms: "How long. . . ." But
suddenly I lose hold of everything I wanted to ask. *To lose the
thread.* What is happening? [pp. 183-184].

As we see in Beutler's account, the period when the cancer advances presents the greatest problem for the patient, her family, the physician, and professional personnel. It is apparent to all that the initial treatment did not eradicate the disease and that progression and infiltration—in other words, metastasis—has set in. The patient changes; she sees and feels the new symptoms, but she is often afraid to visit the doctor and often delays further consultation. As the initial hope for cure diminishes, the patient loses trust in the doctor and in the medical treatment offered. The fear of isolation, separation, and loss becomes overwhelming.

CHANGING OF DOCTOR–PATIENT RELATIONSHIP

One of the most difficult features of this phase is the slow, insidious change that occurs in the doctor–patient relationship. They are no longer partners; the patient suddenly measures and guards his feelings. In this advanced stage, there is a discrepancy between what patients want to know and to whom they pose their questions. Most patients no longer ask the doctor about their medical status, even when the doctor makes a conscious effort to pave the way for them to do so. The patients now realize more fully how dependent they are on the physician's treatment proposals, and at the same time they deeply fear abandonment (Meerwein, 1985a). In the advanced stage of illness, patients end each visit with the sole hope that the doctor will want to see them again, a confirmation of hope: if treatment is still possible, then there is yet a chance that the disease may be counteracted.

The doctor also becomes less secure in his relation with his patient. Even though he may have been truthful at the beginning, he may now start to use selective denial, communicating half-truths to the patient. He rationalizes by claiming concern that the patient might break down or commit suicide were he to know the whole truth. This danger is not always real; if there is open, ongoing communication among patient, oncologist, and treatment team, then the danger of suicide is relatively small. Often the doctor's fear is a projection of his own feelings of powerlessness and self-devaluation onto the patient (Meerwein, 1984).

Only after the patient is confident of the doctor's truthfulness, and after he feels assured of the doctor's continued presence and availability, can he trust again and accept the new therapeutic measures. This new kind of contact with the doctor and treatment team can become a source of the hope for which the patient has waited impatiently.

Alice James, the invalid sister of the novelist Henry and the psychologist William James, contracted breast cancer at the age of 43. In her diary, written almost 100 years ago, she conveys the intensity of her need to find comfort in the doctor-patient relationship after she learned that her breast cancer was terminal. The professional equivocation James (1964) actually receives is the opposite of what she so badly wants and needs:

> January 4, 1892.
> Sir Andrew [doctor] is doubtless good and kind at bottom, but they are all terrible, with that globular manner, talking by the hour without saying anything, while the longing pallid victim stretches out a sickly tendril, hoping for some excrescence, a human wart, to catch on to, but it vainly slips off the polished surface, as comforting and nourishing as that of a billiard ball [p. 226].

Noll (1984) suggests that doctors' behavior is governed more by their need to protect themselves than by their concern for the patient. Noll too longs for the genuine sympathy he does not really get:

> If I will have some more time I will create a typology of medical behaviour and medical personalities. But it is not really necessary, since, on the most important points, they are all essentially similar. They protect themselves not the patient.... For them, personal sympathy for the patient or interest in his individuality is an impossibility. Maybe I am not being fair. How can one possibly have talks with forty patients a day? But I am privileged; all of them talk to me for some time, because of my title [Professor of Law at Zurich University] and out of curiosity, because they found it unusual for someone to reject so quickly the usual treatment methods [p. 45].

Diggelmann (1979) is precise in expressing his need for candid communication unimpeded by the doctor's pretenses or defenses:

> The task of the physician is to understand his specialty so thoroughly that he can with the help of his imagination transform it and so make it comprehensible and accessible to the patient. He must not hide behind professional language and think that his special knowledge is in any case inaccessible to the layman. Imagination has something to do with modesty....
> I believe the patient's fear equals the doctor's.
> The doctor fears the patient, because he thinks that the patient expects too much of him [pp. 108–109].

Diggelmann lays out the patient's need for wisdom, empathy, and imagination on the part of his doctor and stresses the role of clear, honest communication in the cancer patient's recovery:

> A doctor really has to think like a writer, like a poet. He has to look at the patient, he has to talk to him, for hours if necessary. He has to get to know him, he has to examine him as well as possible, and he has to tell him a story, his story, the patient's story. A great deal must be included in this story: the patient's statements, the results of the medical exams, the doctor's knowledge and experience, and, most important, the doctor's life experience, fears, and his capacity to bear failure. He will teach this story to the patient and tell him: if you trust me then I invite you to be my patient. You will help me and you won't forget the story I just told you about your condition and your illness. You will correct me in the course of treatment, you will suddenly interrupt me and say: But Doctor, you said earlier. . . . and I will not deny anything but admit that I forgot. I will repeat comments, correct, and I will reinterpret them and add them to our medical records. That's how we will work together. I will listen to you and you will listen to me and that's how you will become healthy because you want to become healthy. In this way doctor and patient will be one unit. The tighter the union, the better the chance for recovery [pp. 110–111].

The tighter the union between doctor and patient, the better the chance for recovery or, if recovery is not possible, the more the patient feels contained and the better he can approach death with a minimum of anxiety.

In her poem, "Searching for Me," Gitanjali describes the opposite of Diggelmann's trusting relationship to the doctor. By not sharing the fact of her impending death with his young patient, Gitanjali's doctor forfeited her trust and could no longer give her his support. As the dying girl describes it, she, her doctor, and her father all bear a heavy burden, but each is alone, isolated in the knowledge of her impending death. The patient suffers most in this emotional isolation:

Searching for Me

Disillusioned
Discouraged
Despair writ

On his face
The doctor
Holds my hand
Not my attention
He retreats
The moment
I catch his glance
He hurriedly
Looks away.
Neither he, nor my daddy
Can fool me no way
It's poor Mom
Who is lost to the world
And relies heavily on God
Little does she realize
I don't even have
A lean chance.

—

Gitanjali (in Badruddin, 1982, pp.
138–139).

Abba Kovner, the Israeli poet, was hospitalized in New York's
Memorial Sloan Kettering Cancer Center for treatment of his neck tumor
during the progressed stage of his illness. He was very much in need of a
supportive relationship and in the following poem tells us of being
deprived of the contact he needed. In his case, the loneliness and
alienation engendered by the distance and uncommunicativeness of the
medical staff were exacerbated by his being a foreigner, in strange
surroundings, and whose physicians did not know him:

In Their Infuriating Confidence

In the infuriating confidence of the Memorial doc-
     tors
There is something of the mystery of
The mountains of Jerusalem.
—You're just passersby, that's all!
Say the mountains of Jerusalem:
Move on.
Move on.
To the edge of
Border
     Ahead!
Dangerous turn.

Warning!
Slow down!
Slow down.

They come in. They go out.
Walk on.
Walking on
Nothing worse
Than a corridor in the middle of
Laughter—
On. On!

Road cutting through
Samaria;
Sloan-Kettering
Corridor
Cutting through life.
            —Kovner (1988b, p. 3, translated from
              Hebrew by Barbara and Benjamin
              Harshav)

An unempathic, impersonal doctor-patient relationship is especially hard when the patient is in the progressed stage of the illness. Foreigners are not the only ones likely to receive particularly little support at this stage. Doctors who become ill are also unlikely to receive the support of their professional colleagues, who overidentify with, and thus very strongly fear, their sickness. Dr. Stoudemire (1983), a psychiatrist and cancer patient, explains this special situation:

> There was no question that this particular oncologist had a need to avoid me, which was probably a consequence of his over-identification with me. He could not let himself get too "close" to me and pushed far away thoughts of me as a cancer victim. I responded to his efforts at distancing and lack of support with angry resentment and bitterness. . . .
> When one physician treats another, the issue of role reversal is almost impossible to overcome completely. The problem is especially intense if identifications occur and the denial is shared. The treating physician sees too much of his own vulnerability reflected in his colleague, fears it, and denies it. The sick colleague may be approached with excessive defer-ence and treated as if he or she were not "really" a patient. . . .
> The nature of this complicated relationship depends on the mutual identifications and unconscious interplay between the

physicians involved. Some doctors were able to treat me as an ordinary patient—thoroughly, carefully, objectively and empathically. Because of my own resistance to the patient role, I was obviously a difficult patient to treat [p. 383].

On the other hand, as empathic and responsive as the treating physician may be, the patient is almost always ambivalent about him, resentful of his dependence on the doctor, and prone to identifying him as the source of the painful treatment.

Lest this chapter leave the one-sided impression that all physicians are self-protective and distant, unwilling or unable to give cancer patients the warmth they badly need, I would like to end with two statements to the contrary. One is by Reimann (1984), who formed a loving, supportive relationship to her surgeon that lasted till the end of her life:

Professor Gummel was like a father to me. A big surgeon who was capable of keeping his goodness and sympathy. Or did he gain it in the course of the years? Can a human being afford this kind of growing sense of sympathy the more he is confronted with suffering and dying? [p. 334].

The other is by Stewart Alsop (1973) about his physician, John Glick. Their excellent relationship continued unimpeded through the course of most of Alsop's treatment: "I was touched when John said, as he was about to leave, that he had been so worried about that first reading of the marrow that he had had stomach cramps and slept badly. Doctors are people too" (p. 185). Alsop's relationship to Dr. Glick had by this time developed into a close friendship. The young doctor often visited Alsop's home and tended to the patient's medical and psychological needs. Alsop's closeness to his young, intelligent, strong, healthy doctor, who must have represented creativity and life for him, was so strong that Glick's impending departure for a new job made Alsop think of "bowing out":

The thought has occurred to me quite often in recent weeks that perhaps this is a good time to bow out. No doubt it was the state of Alsop, far more than the state of the nation, that caused this thought to occur to me so often. The fact is that I have been depressed, the more so because John Glick, on whom I have become excessively dependent, leaves in a few weeks to take up a new post in California. Moreover, I have been feeling lousy [p. 229].

7

Terminal Phase of Cancer as Described by the Cancer Patient

Ralph
My brother
visits me
in dreams.
Stop visiting,
I say.
He stands
in my dreams
with his wry smile.
I tell him he is
dead. He smiles:
no doubt the irony is
too apparent.
I throw him
to the floor,
stab him
with a fork.
Once, twenty years ago,
I threw him
after I'd seen
my first wrestling
match, waited
for his inevitable
wrestling with me.
Detente.

I ask him to show me
death. He takes my hand,
leads down the tunnel
of trees on dandelion
studded grass.
I hesitate.
If I go,
can I return?
He shakes his head.
I shake mine.
                    —Webster (1980, p. 9)

A life-threatening illness like cancer constitutes a crisis that forces the patient to make a variety of psychic adaptations; the terminal phase can be seen as the height of this crisis. As Webster's poem demonstrates, this crisis cannot be resolved in an ordinary way. There is really no solution to the ambivalence expressed by a suffering patient who clings to life yet yearns for peace and an end to his or her pain.

The threats implicit in cancer—of the unknown and uncertain, of the loss of close family and friends, of the disruption of bodily functions and of identity—all reach their apex in the terminal phase and are a serious threat to the patient's psychic balance. The terminal phase of cancer incorporates the loss of everything that human life contains. The dying patient must mourn everything he knows and loves, and he does not know what to expect in their place.

The terminal phase, as the following passage from Hauri (1982) demonstrates, does not always occur within a strictly defined time:

January 9th, 1980
   The dying started. I can feel it in the way I act with others and others with me. Brothers and sister want to see me once again, to have me with them. They are in a hurry to visit me. Then again a change, improvement, but for how long and for what? I make contact again with friends, communicate with them. Tell them about my pain which nobody can ever feel [p. 69].

When confronted with death in the terminal stage, the patient usually oscillates between acceptance and denial of death. Many patients exhibit extraordinary psychic strength and resourcefulness, as the following quotation by Ted Rosenthal (1973), a late '60s flower child, demonstrates:

There's something about dying that separates you from all other people. Nobody can come to terms with death. Nobody can walk into death and walk back out the same person. Everybody else, no matter who they are, whether they are a poet, a man of power, a frightened little child, whoever it is, they are afraid of the limitless possibilities of their own nature. Once you have nothing, you can be anything, and that's a feeling of freedom [p. 28].

Similar stamina is exhibited in the diary entries of Alice James (1964), written (or when she was too weak, dictated to her life-long companion, Katharine Peabody) during the last three years of her life:

May 31st, 1891

[The doctor said] that a lump that I have had in one of my breasts for three months, which has given me a great deal of pain, is a tumour, that nothing can be done for me but to alleviate pain, that it is only a question of time, etc. This with a delicate embroidery of "the most distressing case of nervous hyperaesthesia" added to a spinal neurosis that has taken me off my legs for seven years; with attacks of rheumatic gout in my stomach for the last twenty, ought to satisfy the most inflated pathologic vanity. It is decidedly indecent to catalogue oneself in this way, but I put it down in a scientific spirit, to show that though I have no productive worth, I have a certain value as an indestructible quantity. . . .

To anyone who has not been there, it will be hard to understand the enormous relief of Sir A.C.'s [doctor] uncompromising verdict, lifting us out of the formless vague and setting us within the very heart of sustaining concrete. One would naturally not choose such an ugly and gruesome method of progression down the Dark Valley of the Shadow of Death. . . . Having it to look forward to for a while seems to double the value of the event, for one becomes suddenly picturesque to oneself, and one's wavering little individuality stands out with a cameo effect and one has the tenderest indulgence for all the abortive little stretchings out which crowd in upon the memory.

I cannot make out whether it is an entire absence or an excess of humor in Destiny to construct such an elaborate exit for my thistle-down personality, especially at this moment when so many of the great of the earth are gobbled up in a day or two by a microbe [pp. 207–209].

James's lines, with their laughter and fear of death, their renunciation and protest, reflect a very individual style of approaching the terminal phase.

Certain features of the terminal phase may facilitate the patient's slow adjustment to impending death. One, as described in the following statement by Alsop (1973), is the patient's growing weakness as his illness progresses:

> In short, for people who are sick, to be a bit sicker—sick unto death itself—holds far fewer terrors than for people who feel well. Both Cy Sulzberger and Bill Attwood [friends] wrote me letters in which they referred to death as the Greek god, Thanatos. It was at this point that I began to think of death as Uncle Thanatos. When I felt sick enough, I even felt a certain affection for Thanatos, and much less fear of him than I had before [p. 134]

"Uncle Thanatos" loses some of his threat for Alsop as Alsop's physical strength fades and after he has been separated from his physician, to whom he has become closely attached:

> I have lived, in short, what John Glick [his physician] calls "a normal life."
> But it has not been altogether normal. It is not normal to wake up every night just before dawn, with a fever of 101 or so, take a couple of pills, and settle down to sweat like a hog for four or five hours. It is not normal to feel so weak you can't play tennis or go trout fishing. And it is not normal either to feel a sort of creeping weariness and a sense of being terribly dependent, like a vampire, on the blood of others. After eight weeks of this kind of "normal" life, the thought of death loses some of its terrors.
> But the most important reason why I felt no panic fear last Saturday was, I think, the strange, unconscious, indescribable process which I have tried to describe in this book—the process of adjustment whereby one comes to terms with death. A dying man needs to die, as a sleepy man needs to sleep, and there comes a time when it is wrong, as well as useless, to resist [p. 299].

In other words, the very losses that make the terminal phase of cancer so fearful may help patients come to terms with impending death. In a terrible way, this can be seen in the following poem by Helen Webster, which describes the American poet's sad surrender to death in the overmechanized, overtechnologized hospital where excretions are treasured more than human warmth:

In The Hospital

I am safe,
stripped to bone.
My orifices
reverenced;
my excretions
treasured.
I am bone clean.
Surrender is easy here.
Death is simple
behind closed doors.
                    —Webster (1980, p. 46)

More fortunate patients in the terminal phase find comforts that protect them from being overwhelmed by the fear of death. Alsop (1973) is sustained by the affectionate care of his family and the feeling that his dead mother and sister are awaiting him "on the other side":

> Mother, Sis said, had asked for a little chat with God. She had told God that she did not want her son Stew or her daughter Corinne to join her in heaven yet; she would tell Him when the time had come. God, of course, had agreed to put off the reunion [p. 34].

Michele Murray, the Washington writer who died of cancer when she was 40, approached death with equanimity by dwelling on the rich emotional life she had had and which she claimed could not be denied her:

Death Poem

What will you have when you finally have me?
Nothing.
Nothing I have not already given
freely each day I spent
not waiting for you
but living
as if the shifting shadows of grapes
and fine-pointed leaves in the shelter
of the arbor would continue to tremble
when my eyes were absent
in memory of my seeing,
or the books fall open where I marked them

when my astonishment overflowed
at a gift come unsummoned, this love
for the open hands of poems,
earth fruit, sun soured grass, the steady
outward lapping stillness of midnight
snowfalls, an arrow of light waking me
on certain mornings with sharp wound
so secret that not even you
will have it when you have me.
You will have my fingers
but not what they touched. Some gestures
outflowing from a rooted being, the memory
of morning light cast on a bed
where two lay together—
the shining curve of flesh!—
they will forever be out of your reach
whose care is with the husks.
                    —Murray (1974, p. 97)

Her memory of fusion with another person, be it in the act of love between a man and a woman or between a mother and child, protects Murray from the all-encompassing fear of death.

Rosenthal (1974) is protected from the fear of death by his sense of unity with nature as he returns to his beloved mountains of California in the terminal phase of his illness. "We're walking home now," he writes, as he contemplates his fusion with nature in death:

O people, I am so sorry.
Nothing can be hid.
It's a circle in the round.
It's group theater,
no wings, no backstage, no leading act.
O, I am weeping, but it's stage center for all of us.
Hide in the weeds but come out naked.
Dance in the sand while lightning bands all around
        us.
Step lightly, we're walking home now.
The clouds take every shape.
We climb up the boulders; there is no plateau.
We cross the stream and walk up the slope.
See, the hawk is diving.
The plain stretches out ahead, then the hills, the
        valleys, the meadows.

Keep moving people. How could I not be among
you?
—Rosenthal (1973, p. 74).

Death is more difficult to face for patients who do not have such consolations and is even worse when they feel deprived of the particular human contact they urgently need. In the next three poems by the dying adolescent Gitanjali, we see how difficult her dying is made, despite her strong faith in God. Each of the poems represents a different phase in Gitanjali's longing for her absent father, who she fears might come too late. His arrival symbolizes for the adolescent girl close union with him as she experienced it in childhood.

Don't Be So Late

I know not
How long I have to wait
Before you decide
To keep the promise you made
To return to my longing arms
Arms that may raise no more
To welcome you
Because they are dying
For lack of strength.

The feeling of isolation
And loneliness which I felt
When I last kissed you goodbye
Has swept over me afresh
I tremble at the thought
Of not seeing you again
Don't be so late
To visit me my Papa dear!
For raise me you will never
From the Dust!

.   .   .   .   .   .

Death is just at the corner
Waiting to sting me
While my gaze is hazy
And fading ever more
The hope is still flickering
To see you

Walk through the door.
When many people
Will throng the way
On the way
To my last journey
Silently shedding tears in pity
Showering me with profound love
And flowers
I wonder if you will be
Amongst them
Silently walking behind me
Or resting my coffin on your shoulders
Where once you carried me
To give me a joy-ride
When I was a child
　　　　　　　—Gitanjali (in Badruddin, 1982, pp.
　　　　　　　108-109).

Gitanjali hopes for a sign of love from her absent father, something to take with her when she needs to go.

Your Message

My eyes are
glued,
Under the
Door.
Wherefrom
Your message
Will come.

In a feverish
Response,
I'll grab
The letter,
And hold it
Against
My throbbing
Heart.

What you have to
Say,
Is up to you.
What my eyes will

Scan for,
Is up to me
—Gitanjali (in Badruddin, 1982, p. 135)

Still waiting, but too badly disappointed that he does not arrive, Gitanjali prophesies her father's future, which is colored by her understandable anger.

The Pain of Repentance

you will
at last
need me
want me
sometime
in life.

you will
I'm sure
call out
for me
when
lonesome
some-night.
but, alas!
all you will
find is the . . .
dreary silence.

in tears
with fear
in dread
instead of
love.
you will
wish me
near.
but,
I'm sorry
I'll be by then
long gone
wherefrom
no one
ever returns.

the pain
of
repentance
will soak you
in grief and
guilt, and
endless sorrow
is all that . . .
you will reap.
for all the
heartache
that was mine
because
to me,
you were
unkind.

my eyes though
dull
still flicker
with love.
in them
you will find
yet,
no anger
nor hate.

come, oh! please come!
come and see—
my pitiful sight,
I who once
not so long ago
was your . . .
cherished child

> —Gitanjali (in Badruddin, 1982, pp.
> 140-141).

The dying patient faces emotional problems of great magnitude, including the fear of death, the fear of the painful ordeal of dying, and the devastating fear of abandonment. The terror of dying is described by Reimann (1984), who is plagued in her last days by nightmares of her death:

Interrupted again. Early morning. A new try. This awful "cancerness" has lots of consequences that I hadn't imagined, and I was unprepared for. What I was not prepared for: the horrible dreams each night, the fear of death, which never leaves me, the feeling of a provisional life, the lack of pleasure, and the inability to plan ahead more than till the day after tomorrow or the following week. Something really changed. One can see nothing of physical lack, my early inculcated Prussian posture now comes to the fore and nobody would think that I am damaged or even ill. What slowly but surely kills me is the fear, panic, horror (worse, on the other hand, the fearlessness that comes of indifference). Professor Gummel told me at the time that the cells can turn malignant . . . ; Since then I think that sometimes, or even soon, the next round will start. This word "susceptibility" grows exuberantly and eats me up, and if I can't find a way to free myself from it I will go crazy or commit suicide because I can't bear the fear and the waiting [p. 298].

Psychologically, the terminal phase is initiated when the doctor is forced to tell his patient that medical treatment will no longer arrest or cure the disease and that he can give only palliative care to relieve symptoms and diminish pain. Most of our literary examples describe the very beginning of this phase, because later the patient typically withdraws into himself and no longer feels the need to communicate his feelings in writing.

The entire doctor–patient relationship in the terminal phase is colored by the patient's impending death. The approach that the doctor and treatment team take at this stage is vital. A great deal of understanding and tact is required of them if they are to help the patient as he approaches his end. On one hand, consensus in the healing community holds it desirable to encourage patients to verbalize their concerns and feelings about death. On the other hand, many doctors prefer to avoid such discussions at all costs. Neither approach serves the best interests of the patient.

The imminence of death is very obvious in the terminal phase. The terminal cancer patient knows that he is dying without being reminded of it. There is usually little comfort for the patient at this late stage in discussing his impending death when it is so close and so plain. Far from bringing relief, clumsy efforts by the treatment team to get the patient to discuss his feelings about the subject constitute pressure and cause emotional discomfort. The dying patient's need to avoid forced reminders of death is illustrated in Reimann's (1984) apology for not attending the funeral of her aunt, of whom she had been fond:

Under psychological pressure I have become shy of everything having to do with death. Maybe you think this is cruel
since she is an aunt who I used to like to visit very much. But
it's self-protection. I only have to imagine the atmosphere of
the cemetery and I start crying. Sorry that I'm talking so much
about myself but I can't get over my story, I can't show it to
anybody else [p. 301].

Not wanting to be at a cemetery or attend a funeral is a form of
self-protection. Similarly, in the terminal phase of illness, most patients
prefer not to be inundated with flowers from well-meaning friends or
bombarded with letters of sympathy. Such well-meaning activities only
make the patient feel closer to death, buried and mourned while still alive.

On the other hand, what Cassileth and Cassileth (1982) term the "new
conspiracy of silence" that develops in this phase is no better. When
family and treatment team are unable or unwilling to admit to the patient
that they know he is dying, the patient is forced to deal alone with the
magnitude of the situation and the terrible fears and sadness that attend it.
Consequently he feels utterly abandoned. Silence deprives patients of the
opportunity to ventilate their fears and share their anxieties if they wish to
and contributes to the fear of abandonment which, along with the fear of
pain, is the dying patient's dominant concern, as we will see in the next
chapter.

The following quotation from Hauri (1982), who recognizes the
doctor's dilemma at this stage, points to the dying patient's need for the
doctor's concern, tact, tacit understanding, and, as always in cancer, gentle,
honest answers:

The doctor didn't tell me that I'll recover, he told me that I
will die.

The doctor, his office, the hated way to him. The talk in
those pictureless white rooms, neon lights on the ceiling,
glittering metal. I pound him with questions and he answers
between the lines, between door and hinges with a special
tone in his voice. In the way he wishes me merry Christmas, in
his look, in his patience. He brings warmth into these cold
rooms, he fills them up, he is patient, he knows that one needs
to be patient with cancer patients. He takes enough time; he
makes it a principle. He is happy when I feel a little better.
There is a sense of urgency about him; we are both given over
to concern; he sees the limits of his art, how the cancer
changes my body, how it grows exuberantly, expands, hits.

Sometimes he uses "medical distance" to avoid my uncomfortable questions, sometimes he pretends that he doesn't know but shows that he knows more than he wants to tell. A doctor sometimes is also a human being. A great deal is coming up in me now. I could vomit. At least I cry [p. 71].

When the illness is terminal, the patient's sense of alienation may mount to profound loneliness. Conversation between the one who knows that his time is running out and the one who has unlimited time is very difficult, says Noll (1984): "Conversation stops not at death but much earlier. Understanding is missing" (p. 87). Kubler-Ross's (1969) stages—denial, anger, bargaining, depression, and acceptance—are often mistakenly considered to follow each other in an inflexible sequence. The stages, however, are not all invariable or even typical of all dying patients, and one sometimes finds all five stages in a single interview. The terminal phase is frequently more difficult for the observer, since the patient usually withdraws into himself as life draws to a close. The constant presence of others can help the patient and family cope during the remaining period.

In this stage, the patient's dependency needs overflow to the paramedical personnel. The almost total dependence of the terminally ill patient is accompanied, in some cases, by intense frustration and humiliation, especially for those who previously led independent lives and made their own decisions. With empathic care, these tensions can be verbalized and diminished, and the patient can regress to a childlike existence where others attend to his or her physical needs. Then communication often becomes minimal, especially in the area of the patient's anxieties. Most patients display withdrawal or detachment, which can be a positive sign as they prepare themselves for death. Silence becomes the language of this last phase. "The challenge is less what to say than how to listen," observe Cassileth and Cassileth (1982, p. 110).

At this late point, patients do not want to talk about death or dying, because this brings them closer to the inevitable. A patient who is sick enough to die knows it without being told. At the end patients often come to accept the inevitable result of their illness without great anxiety. Sometimes their chief concern is for the future care of their children. Closer to death, however, they often become increasingly more detached from the realities of life and will even stop asking about the children. It is a time when the patient's active coping strategies change into passive cooperation.

Because the patient feels lonely in the experience of impending death, which cannot be shared with anybody, the presence and support of the nurses is crucial. Nursing care—bathing the patient and attending to other personal needs—becomes immensely important. In this last stage, patients often feel that they are untouchable. Touching, holding hands, washing and massaging the body, are all ways to give a quiet message of consolation.

The nursing team and the family also take over the patient's ego functions at this time. Sometimes they have to act and talk for him, since he may no longer be able to speak himself. An example that comes to mind is a 24-year-old terminally ill cancer patient whom I treated for many years until his death. At our last session, this once very active patient was too weak to write the date of our next meeting in his diary and softly asked me to do it for him, an attempt to reassure my presence also the next day.

Oral needs like hunger and thirst should be attended to empathically, and a program to fight pain must be organized. The program of care and nurturing can awaken in the patient memories of past "good objects" (like the mother's breast); these good objects then become a pillar against the intrusion of the "bad parts," represented by the cancer (Meerwein, 1985a).

Gitanjali hoped to return in death to the deep, protected sleep of childhood:

An Appeal

Death
Who are you?
Where do you come from?
Where will you take me?
Is the way long?
Is it too dark?

I do claim to be brave
And yet am afraid
For I know not
What's beyond.
Death
I do some times
Expect you
And at times hope
You'd never come
If you must take me
Do be merciful
Take me where no one can hurt me
Or cause me pain
And I have an appeal
Do please be kind

> And let me sleep . . .
> As in my childhood I did
> —Gitanjali (in Badruddin, 1982, p. 34).

"Death I do sometimes expect you and . . . hope you'd never come,"— these two contradictory thoughts are what we often find when we care for the dying cancer patient.

In the terminal phase, the cancer patient often shows a kind of inner psychic splitting, which facilitates his acceptance of impending death. Two opposite ideas are verbalized: one, a full realization of the closeness of death; the other, a faith in surviving, often expressed in vivid fantasies about the future. The perception of this split and the psychological handling of it is, for those surrounding the patient, extremely difficult, since the split stands in opposition to the reality principle that governs our ordinary, day-to-day existence. The irrationality that this split communicates to us seems to go against our understanding of reality (Dreifuss and Meerwein, 1984b).

With the help of this split the patient overcomes his fear of death and so can still remain in communication with his environment, the premature loss of which profoundly threatens him. People who would like to accompany the cancer patient to the end of life need to understand this split. If they refuse to make the split themselves, either by refusing to accept the patient's fantasies of the future or by denying the reality of the patient's impending death, they cannot be partners on the path that the patient must walk. They have to be able to deal simultaneously with both parts of the patient, the dying one and the surviving one. Only then does the dying human being feel contained as a whole human being who can receive loving care for both his surviving and dying parts.

Wander (1980), close to her death, illustrates this split quite clearly. She writes in a letter:

> What did I want to tell you? How the borders in us between pain, despair and pleasure can interflow. From the deepest feeling of apathy and abandonment I fall without transitions into an euphoric mood. All life compresses into a tiny little room, so much so that it presses on the walls and the room explodes and expands. In the process I am flooded with light (Angels in chariots of fire . . .). I laugh again, splash happiness and mockery and make the doctors and nurses laugh. The other women patients look at me in disbelief, some envious, angry, without understanding. Some come and look into my eyes, as if they want to drink from them [p. 260].

Reimann (1984), in the terminal phase of her breast cancer, describes her counterdepressive reaction to a day at hospital spent crying out of loneliness, pain, and frustration:

> I would like to do a thousand crazy things, when I get out of here [the hospital]; to stumble through a thousand bars and dance on their counters, to sow flowers, to write my book and to kiss a whole lot of men and to drive my car very fast [p. 319].

Reimann never left the hospital.

Rosenthal (1973) also describes the "positive" side of the split in the terminal phase:

> I realized in fact that I felt really good for the first time in my life. Not just a flash of good feeling like twenty minutes of good feeling, but a sustained feeling that I had nothing, and having nothing I had nothing to lose, and having nothing to lose I could be anything. I didn't have a self-image to worry about. And not having a self-image to worry about meant I had no definition. I had nothing I had to be, nothing I had to care about. And I felt free. I felt as if I could leap out the window, not out of despair or fear, but just for the hell of it, just for the fun of it [p. 27].

The terminal cancer patient strives to give meaning to his life. Often he finds this meaning in the possibility of surviving in the memory of the people close to him as a good, loving, and creative human being. He would like to resolve his negative feelings toward his past, toward his family and friends, and himself, so as to approach his end in a conflict-free way. The terminal cancer patient needs help in mourning his body and his outside world, thereby regaining his good, inner experiences and fantasies. The following poems by the Swiss poet Ruth Reichstein, who suffered from terminal breast cancer, show the strong impetus in this direction:

Michaelis	*Michaelis*
An	On
einem	a
Spinnen-	spider
faden haengt	thread hangs
das letzte Licht	the last light
	—Reichstein (1988, p. 53)

Trost	Consolation
An den	On the
kahlen Laerchen	bare larches
Zaepfchen	cones
Immer zwei	always two
beieinander	side by side

—Reichstein (1988, p. 42)

It is the patient's move from her external world to her inner fantasies that will sustain her as she crosses to the other world.

8

"The Death of Ivan Ilych" —Pain and Its Relief in Terminal Cancer

Fear of pain is a prevalent concern for cancer patients. Many cancer patients fear that as the illness progresses they will have to suffer devastating pain without adequate relief. Pain makes them feel powerless, and they experience it as endless. Memories of pain-free periods or the hope of a pain-free future cannot bring relief.

About 60% of all terminal cancer patients experience severe pain, and possibly a third of these die with their pain unrelieved (Twycross, 1980). The incidence of pain varies with the primary site of the tumor. Pain is relatively unusual in leukemia and lymphoma but is common in a high percentage of primary bone tumors (85%), in cancer of the buccal cavity (80%), and in genitourinary cancers (male: 75%; female: 70%) (Twycross, 1984b).

Because of its prevalence, pain and its relief play a dominant role in patients' thoughts about cancer and are critical for the psychological guidance of both cancer patients and their treatment teams. Since pain manifests itself mostly in the progressed or terminal phase of cancer, there are few references to pain in the literary works of cancer patients. Instead, I take as my example Tolstoy's (1882) short story, "The Death of Ivan Ilych," which deals with the intense emotional stresses and physical sufferings of a 45-year-old magistrate during the last three months of his fatal illness. Although Tolstoy never names the protagonist's disease, C. Schein (1981), Chief Surgeon of the Albert Einstein College of Medicine, has retrospectively diagnosed Ivan Ilych's illness as cancer and extrapolated from Tolstoy's account the differential diagnosis of a carcinoma of the body of the pancreas.

Tolstoy's vivid, detailed description of his fictitious patient, Ivan Ilych, and of the evolution of Ilych's pain allows us to delineate the different components of the pain terminal cancer patients typically suffer. First, a short "anamnesis" of Ivan Ilych: "Ivan Ilych's life had been most simple and most ordinary and therefore most terrible," writes Tolstoy (1882, p. 104). Ivan Ilych graduated from law school, then went to the provinces to find an agreeable position where he served for five years. Then he was offered the post as an examining magistrate, giving him a lot of power, which, the author stresses, he never abused. After settling in this new town he met his future wife, Praskovya Fedorovina Milchel, who became pregnant and soon "began to disturb the pleasure and propriety of their life" (p. 109). After the birth of their first child, Ivan Ilych became more involved in his official work, and his wife grew more irritable. After seven years' service in this town, he was transferred to another province as Public Prosecutor. There his wife was especially unhappy, blaming her husband for every inconvenience. He and his wife now fought frequently, their quarrels punctuated by rare periods of amorousness. After enduring this unsatisfying situation for seven years, Ivan unexpectedly obtained an appointment in his former ministry and also found a delightful house. With much care he decorated this house, planning to surprise his family. One day while mounting a stepladder, he slipped and knocked his side against the knob of a window frame. Ivan Ilych attributes his illness to this accident.

His discomfort begins as a gnawing pain in the side, which he does not initially identify as an illness: "It could not be called ill health if Ivan Ilych sometimes said that he had a queer taste in his mouth and felt some discomfort in his left side" (p. 120). However, "his discomfort increased and, though not exactly painful, grew into a sense of pressure in his side, accompanied by ill humour" (p. 120). Now, for the first time, our patient consults a doctor to investigate the source of his pain:

> From the doctor's summing up Ivan Ilych concluded that things were bad, but that for the doctor, and perhaps for everybody else, it was a matter of indifference, though for him it was bad. And this conclusion struck him painfully, arousing in him a great feeling of pity for himself and of bitterness towards the doctor's indifference to a matter of such importance [p. 122].

When the patient tries to probe his physician as to whether or not his illness is dangerous, the doctor refuses to give him a straight answer. On the way home, Ilych tries to analyze what the doctor had actually said: "Is my condition bad? Is it very bad? Or is there as yet nothing much wrong?" (p. 122). His questions unanswered by his doctor, Ivan becomes depressed and his "ache, this dull gnawing ache that never ceased for a moment, seemed to have acquired a new and more serious significance from the doctor's dubious remarks. Ivan Ilych now watched it with a new and oppressive feeling" (p. 122).

We see from this passage that to be able to fight pain, the patient is fully dependent on the understanding and good will of his doctor. It is thus very important for the doctor to understand the patient's pain and its meaning and the different techniques of pain relief, both medical and psychological. To fight the patient's pain, the doctor must make a precise pain diagnosis, a so-called anamnesis of pain. To judge from the story of our fictive patient, Ivan Ilych's first pain anamnesis would be: this pain is first associated with rapid weight loss, irritability, pronounced depression, inability to concentrate at work. It is aggravated by eating: "His bursts of temper always came just before dinner, often just as he began to eat his soup" (p. 120).

Pain is a dual phenomenon consisting of both the patient's perception of the sensation and his psychological reaction to that sensation. One's pain threshold varies according to one's mood and his morale. Important factors that modulate pain are anxiety, depression, and fatigue. Explaining to patients the mechanisms underlying pain often reduces anxiety, and showing continuous concern for them raises morale (Twycross and Ventafridda 1980). Ignoring mental and social factors when treating pain may result in an otherwise relievable pain's remaining unameliorated.

Cancer can cause pain in any part of the body and through a wide variety of mechanisms. Patients often put on a brave face for the doctor, so even if they have severe pain they may not look distressed. Moreover, by itself a patient's account does not always enable the physician to reach an accurate assessment of the intensity of the pain. As Noll (1984) says, "My pain is present, blunt, and heavy, but I cannot talk about it, because I cannot relate it to any experience I ever had in the past" (p.236). The doctor must also know what drugs have failed to relieve the patient in the past, whether his sleep is disturbed, and in what way his activity has become limited. In addition, the patient's spouse, or another close family member, should be interviewed for a complete picture. All these pieces of information should be taken into account. If the patient says, "It's all pain, doctor," he is telling us not only that the pain is severe and overwhelming, but also that it is compounded by anxiety, depression, and loss of morale.

Ivan Ilych's loss of morale was, in part, due to his physicians' lack of empathy, their deceiving him about what his disease really was, and to the lack of sympathy, even hostility, of his wife and colleagues at work. Praskovya Fidorovna's attitude toward her husband's illness was that it was his own fault. When Ivan Ilych tried to communicate his fear to her, she did not really listen, though she told him to take his prescribed medicine regularly. This he did, but his pain did not diminish. At work, Ivan felt that the people "were watching him inquisitively as a man whose place might soon be vacant" (p. 126). All in all, he was in greatest pain when he quarreled with his wife, had problems in his official work, or was unlucky at cards. He consulted yet more doctors but soon lost confidence in their treatment as well, and "the pain in his side oppressed him and seemed to grow worse and more incessant, while the taste in his mouth grew stranger and stranger" (p. 125). He lost his appetite and strength. Far from reassuring him, the reactions he encountered from his wife and colleagues confirmed his worst suspicions: "[Ivan] was not deceiving himself; something terrible, new, and more important than anything before in his life, was taking place within him of which he alone was aware" (p. 125).

Pain isolates the patient in his already lonely dying. He realizes that for the medical community pain is part of the daily routine. For him, however, pain is new, overwhelming, shameful, something that takes over his entire life. Ivan felt that his life was poisoned and was poisoning the lives of others and that this poison did not relent, but instead penetrated more and more deeply into his whole being. With this awareness and with physical pain accompanying the terror, he must go to bed, often to lie awake the greater part of the night.

Ivan Ilych's pain exacerbates his anxiety to the point of terror. His emotions reach this extreme because he has no one with whom to share his great anxiety as he gradually acknowledges that he must be terminally ill and close to death. Both doctor and family avoid discussing his illness and future and therefore push him into an abyss of loneliness and terror that further elevates his physical suffering. Every time he thinks that things might be looking up, he feels again the "old familiar dull, gnawing pain, stubborn and serious" (p. 129), which makes him realize that "it is a question of life and death" (p. 129). As Tolstoy states, "Ivan Ilych saw he was dying and he was in continual despair" (p. 131). Unable to share his fears with his unempathic wife and doctors, "he would go to his study, lie down, and again be alone with *it*: face to face with *it*. And nothing could be done with *it* except to look at it and shudder" (p. 134).

For today's cancer patients the best results are obtained by adopting a broad-spectrum approach to fighting pain, using two or more treatments in combination (Twycross, 1980). The use of analgesics is but one way of elevating the patient's pain threshold (Twycross, 1984). Some patients continue to experience pain, especially when they move about, despite analgesics. Other drugs, including psychotropic ones, as well as radiotherapy and nerve blocks, may thus need to be offered. In this case one should also suggest commonsense modifications in the patient's activities and perhaps intervene to facilitate communication with his family as well.

A 1980 survey of cancer patients in St. Christopher's Hospice in

London estimated that of 100 patients, 82 were in pain (Baines, 1984). For some patients, relief may be obtained fairly easily. With other patients, particularly those who experience pain in movement and those whose pain is compounded by severe anxiety and depression, satisfactory pain relief may take three to four weeks of inpatient treatment to achieve, but it is obtainable nonetheless. In all patients it should be possible to achieve some minimum improvement within 24 to 48 hours. Apart from these broad outlines, I shall not discuss the current medical approaches to cancer pain further save to say that cancer is a progressive pathological process that continually causes new pain to develop or old pain to reemerge. Whenever this happens, the patient's needs should be reassessed. He might require a modification in drug therapy, additional radiation therapy, a nerve-block, a new psychological assessment of his current life situation and its impact on family dynamics, or other interventions. If the pain becomes overwhelming to the patient, he needs to be reassessed within hours.

Hypnosis and self-hypnosis are ways of combatting predictable pain and discomfort, such as the inflammation that typically follows the injection of chemotherapeutic toxins. Similarly, relaxation techniques can be used to combat the pain associated with muscle spasms. The common denominator in these and related techniques is that it allows the patient to control to varying degrees his pain and so diminishes the feeling of helplessness that often accompanies the progression of a malignant process (Portenoy and Foley, 1989).

Without denigrating these techniques and the importance of drugs, Tolstoy emphasizes the human factor in Ivan's pain relief or lack thereof. Because Ivan Ilych's doctor did not take the patient's anxiety and depression into account, the opium and hypodermic injections of morphine the doctor gave him did not provide permanent relief: "The dull depression he experienced in a somnolent condition [owing to the medication] at first gave him a little relief, but only as something new, afterwards it became as distressing as the pain itself or even more so" (p. 135). Ilych's pain was further made worse by the deception of his family, who did not want to admit he was dying:

> What tormented Ivan Ilych most was the deception, the lie, which for some reason they all accepted, that he was not dying, but was simply ill. . . . This deception tortured him—their not wishing to admit what they all knew and what he knew, but wanting to lie to him concerning his terrible condition, and wishing and forcing him to participate in that lie. . . . He wanted to scream: "Stop lying! You know and I know that I am dying. Then at least stop lying about it" [p. 137].

The only relief the suffering patient obtained was from an assistant butler, Gerasim, a clean, fresh, peasant lad who came to his aid. When the patient was compelled to ask for help in cleaning himself, for support so that he would not fall, Gerasim would say: "What's a little trouble? It's a case of illness with you, sir" (p. 130). Gerasim's presence was so comforting that Ivan often did not want to let him leave, especially since everyone else now stayed distant from him so as not to have to admit his dying. Ivan sought relief from this deception as much as from physical pain: "Only Gerasim recognized it and pitied him. And so Ivan Ilych felt at ease only with him" (pp. 137-138). Tolstoy stresses the dying patient's need for genuine human sympathy: "At certain moments after prolonged suffering he wished most of all . . . for someone to pity him as a sick child is pitied. He longed to be petted and comforted" (p. 138). Tolstoy also points out the difficulty the dying person has in asking for that vital sympathy. When left alone, Ivan Ilych "groaned not so much with pain, terrible though that was, as from mental anguish" (p. 140).

Once he entered a new stage in the illness, Ivan Ilych should have received a second pain diagnosis. His new symptoms, loss of appetite and strength, malodorous breath and stool, should have been taken into account. By questioning the patient, the doctors could have learned, as the reader does, that Ivan felt most at ease when he had his legs raised on Gerasim's shoulder, so allowing for a psoas relaxation (Schein, 1981, p. 416). Had his physicians not turned a blind eye, they might have become aware of the intensification of his anger and depression, and, from that, they might also have learned how much his isolation contributed to his pain. Perhaps they might have considered trying to improve the attitude of his wife and daughter.

Tolstoy's description shows clearly that Ivan's pain was only in part a physiological pain. The larger part of it was caused by his intense feeling of loneliness and narcissistic rage. The people around him deliberately chose not to talk openly about his illness and its terminal course. The patient wanted to regress but could do so, to a certain extent, only with his butler, Gerasim, the only one who openly acknowledged that he was dying. The following death fantasy demonstrates how the dying patient's pain is exacerbated by fear and isolation:

> It seemed to him that he and his pain were being thrust into
> a narrow, deep black sack, but though they were pushed
> further and further in they could not be pushed to the bottom.
> And this, terrible enough in itself, was accompanied by suffer-
> ing. He was frightened yet wanted to fall through the sack, he
> struggled but yet cooperated. And suddenly he broke through,
> fell, and regained consciousness. . . . He wept on account of his

helplessness, his terrible loneliness, the cruelty of man, the cruelty of God, and the absence of God [p. 146]

Following this fantasy, the patient became more and more depressed and could no longer leave his sofa. In what one may guess was an attempt to avoid facing his doctors and his wife, he steadfastly turned to the wall. As he neared his end, "Ivan Ilych's physical sufferings were terrible, but worse than the physical sufferings were his mental sufferings, which were his chief torture" (p. 152).

Three days before his death, Ilych began to scream and did not stop until he died. This brings us to the third pain anamnesis. In the final stage of Ivan's illness, his excruciating pain renders him bedridden and makes him scream out without respite. The opium and morphine he is given are of little avail against the torment that his abysmal isolation makes so much worse than it had to have been.

Only a few hours before he dies is Ivan's suffering somewhat alleviated. Relief was brought by his schoolboy son, who crept softly into the room and came up to his bedside. The dying man was still screaming desperately and waving his arms. His hand fell on the boy's head. The boy caught it, pressed it to his lips, and began to cry:

> At that very moment Ivan Ilych fell through and caught sight of the light, and it was revealed to him that though his life had not been what it should have been, this could still be rectified.
>
> . . . .
>
> . . . And suddenly it grew clear to him that what had been oppressing him and would not leave him was all dropping away at once from two sides, from ten sides, and from all sides. . . .
>
> . . . He sought his former accustomed fear of death and did not find it. "Where is it? What death?" There was no fear because there was no death. In place of death there was light [pp. 155-156].

As his son held his hand and guided him to the "narrow deep sack"— or as Noll (1984, p. 74), writes, to the "black hole," the "negative world," the "none world," Ivan let himself fall into it and found light. His life suddenly regained meaning in the union with his son, and death lost its threat.

Today there are precise guidelines and ample studies and published accounts of clinical experiences in fighting and alleviating the pain of terminal cancer patients. And yet patients often do not receive appropriate, individualized treatment to control their pain, for a variety of conscious and unconscious reasons emanating from both doctor and patient. For one, young physicians typically are not well enough educated in the broad-spectrum approach to fighting pain and are reluctant to ask their more experienced colleagues for help. Another bitterly ironic reason is that the prescription of pain control medicine often becomes the only task the doctor can perform in face of the overpoweringly malignant progress of the disease. By keeping the patient in some pain, and thus compelling him to ask for his pain medication, the doctor can maintain an active relationship with the patient in a situation where he has no other medical benefits to offer. Obviously, this motive is not a conscious one (Meerwein, 1985a).

Unconscious defenses may also result in inadequate pain control. For example, the doctor may fear being drawn into a symbiotic union with a dying patient whom drugs have deprived of the full control of his will. The physician is responsible for medicating a largely unconscious human being who is soon to die. The situation calls for the physician to be sensitive to that patient's state, sensitive enough to keep him from pain, and this entails drawing closer to a person who is both dying and unable to speak his own mind. One can well understand that this circumstance can be anxiety provoking. These fears may be intensified by the idea that pain belongs to life and that a state without pain is a state close to death. The doctor may thus unconsciously believe that by letting the patient suffer he can avert the patient's psychic death and thereby avoid becoming enmeshed in a "narcissistic dual union" with him (Meerwein, 1985).

Other unconscious motives in the doctor have a more aggressive character. He might feel a strong resistance to allowing the patient to gain the secondary satisfaction of euphoria entailed in analgesic medicines (Meerwein, 1984). He may withhold proper pain control out of feelings of vengeance toward a difficult or unpleasant patient. He may harbor fantasies that illness, in particular cancer, is self-imposed; and if the treatment does not give the wished-for result, he may rationalize that it is the patient's fault and that pain is the price to be paid (Meerwein, 1984). All these and similar motives are, of course, generally unconscious and stand in opposition to the ethical ideals of the medical profession.

The patient too may have an unconscious interest in being kept in pain despite a sincere conscious wish for pain control. For some patients, controlling the intake of their pain medication often reflects the wish to be able still to control their regression and helplessness, which are products of the malignant progression of the disease. A common fear is that death is likely to come sooner or more suddenly in the somnolent state produced by analgesic pain medicine.

Then, too, there may be a need to maintain alertness and mental clarity. As Noll (1984) asks, "How long can one get rid of pain without influencing one's consciousness?" (p. 258). The patient might have fantasies that his cancer was precipitated by some wrong or sin on his part, in which case unrelieved pain may gratify an unconscious wish for punishment (Meerwein, 1984). Similarly, the isolated patient who feels worthless may try to strengthen his self-worth and defend against a depressive state by masochistically clinging to the pain, feeling sustained only by the struggle to overcome it. Such a patient might even fantasize that pain in this life will be rewarded after death. The treating doctor or therapist must recognize these kinds of masochistic reactions in the patient and disabuse him of such ideas, in order to open the way to adequate pain control and a comfortable dying.

I would like to end this section with the poem that Rainer Maria Rilke wrote in his notebook shortly before his death of chronic leukemia:

> Komm du, du letzter, den ich anerkenne,
> heilloser Schmerz in leiblichen Geweb:
> wie ich im Geiste brannte, sieh, ich brenne
> in dir; das Holz hat lange widerstrebt,
> der Flamme, die du loderst, zuzustimmen,
> nun aber naehr' ich dich und brenn in dir.
> Mein hiesig Mildsein wird in deinem Grimmen
> ein Grimm der Hoelle nicht von hier.
> Ganz rein, ganz planlos frei von Zukunft stieg
> ich auf des Leidens wirren Scheiterhaufen,
> so sicher nirgend Kuenftiges zu kaufen
> um dieses Herz, darin der Vorrat schwieg.
> Bin ich es noch, der da unkenntlich brennt?
> Erinnerungen reiss ich nicht herein.
> O Leben, Leben: Draussensein.
> Und ich in Lohe. Niemand der mich kennt.
>
> Come, then, my last and latest acceptation,
> pain in this fleshly web beyond all cure:
> as once in mind, see now my conflagration
> in you; the wood no longer can abjure
> agreement with that flame which you're outthrow-
>   ing:
> I feed you now and burn in you as well.
> My earth-born mildness in your fury's growing
> a fury not of earth but hell.
> So pure, so planless-free from all to-come,
> I climbed this dizzy faggot-pile of pain,
> so sure I'd nowhere sacrifice, to gain
> a future, all this heart's uncounted sum.
> Am I still that, unrecognizably consumed?

> I snatch no memories inside.
> O living, living: being outside.
> And I in flame. And no one knowing me
> —Rilke (1966, p. 354).

This final poem by Rilke encapsulates the totality of pain for the dying cancer patient.

PART II

Psychoanalytic Perspectives

9

MOURNING, LOSS,

AND

CREATIVITY

In Part I, taking as our frame of reference the disease process and the course of treatment, we looked at the cancer stories from a psychooncological perspective. As we have seen, both the nature of a patient's fears and the optimal responses that can be given to those fears undergo significant changes depending on the current clinical situation. In Part II, we shall be looking at the literary and artistic products of cancer victims from an entirely different perspective. Principally, I will be reporting on my own and others' psychotherapeutic work with seriously ill and terminal cancer patients, work that for the most part is informed by psychoanalytic principles. Moreover, much of what I have to report arises within the relatively specialized confines of art therapy, a discipline with which the reader may be unfamiliar. I hope, however, that what is at stake in these reports is sufficiently universal to be accessible both to the general reader and to professionals from other disciplines.

On entering into this different realm of discussion, we will have to shift our level of analysis. We will not only be adopting a more finely grained look at the data, but we will also be relying on a more subtle interpretive rationale, one that takes as its point of departure not the actual circumstances of the patient, but the inner psychic reality through which those circumstances are understood and mediated. Moreover, in pursuit of an understanding of that psychic reality, we will be concerned with topics that, at first glance, seem far removed from the realities of a hospital bed. The purpose of this chapter is to introduce those topics and to establish, at least in a preliminary way, their special relevance to the dying patient. From there we will go on to see how these themes can be utilized in dealing with cancer patients psychotherapeutically.

None of this is meant to supercede either the psychooncological approach or the vitality of the cancer stories reviewed in the first part of this book. Far from it. If our authors' bravery and their determination to keep at their craft against all odds have accomplished anything, it has been to help us gain insight into both the terrible realities of cancer and the special needs of those who must wrestle with this illness. For that alone, they deserve our admiration and our gratitude.

But there is an entirely different set of questions that can be asked of the cancer literature. These questions have to do with the psychological wellsprings of creativity, with its relation to courage and the ability to persevere, and with its very special relation to the themes of separation, loss, and mourning. These issues become clear only when we extract ourselves from the gripping immediacy of the cancer stories, when we take a measure of intellectual distance from the life-and-death struggles going on within. At first, something within us may rebel at the prospect, as though perspective were tantamount to detachment and both were tantamount to disrespect. Yet, I submit, the questions go to the heart of the human creativity, and they are no less pertinent for being asked in the context of mortality. Nor, I think, would our authors object to our moving to the plane of reflection; if anything, they have been there before us.

Consider, for example, that the stories we have just reviewed are by turns ironic, touching, funny, inspiring, sad, moving. The one thing they are not is depressing. Why is that? How is it that we, as readers, can participate in the experience of ultimate loss without feeling totally overwhelmed by it? What does that tell us about the special power of the creative response? Then, too, consider that the writers themselves were still able to draw on their special gifts in the midst of the most impossible circumstances imaginable. Are theirs the responses of a few unusually courageous persons? Or is there something intrinsic to the nature of creativity that it stands ready to respond in these emergency conditions? Perhaps creativity has some fundamental relation to the problems of separation and loss, problems that reach their apogee with the threat of death but that, in any only relatively lessened form, plague us our whole lives. And if that is the case, might we not further suppose that creativity has a special role to play in the human psyche, that it is, as it were, a special gift from the gods enabling us to negotiate the one thing that uniquely frightens us, our final aloneness?

If a single quality can be said to typify our cancer authors, it is their gift for great moral courage. It is this, I think, which we most admire in their stories. That they were talented and gifted, in ways that most of us are not, seems by comparison to be almost trivial. In contemplating our own mortality, it is not their gifts that we envy in our cancer authors, but their grace and their resolve. Conceivably, however, we misjudge the issue a bit.Perhaps there is something inherent in creativity that enables one to be braver than one otherwise would be. Perhaps if an Alsop or a Gitanjali could return, they would tell us that, no, they did not think themselves unusually brave people, nor did they think they struggled more mightily for their composure than did the people lying in the beds next to them. They just had an urge to write about what they were going through, they might tell us, and somehow that helped. And, just possibly, that puzzled them as much as it should us.

In this chapter, I shall pursue the puzzle of creativity and its special relation to loss in the hope of throwing at least a little light on that subject. In general, I will be drawing on two sources of information, one relatively abstract and the other highly concrete. First, I shall briefly review various psychoanalytic theories about the origins of creativity in human develop- ment, paying particular attention to how it is from the first connected with issues of separation. Second, I shall be drawing from interviews I have conducted with a number of artists and writers who were willing to share with me their private thoughts about how cancer affected their work and how they tried to use their creative abilities to fashion a response to the disease. For their time and for their willingness to share with me the fruits of an ongoing struggle, I am grateful.

To be sure, I intend to draw no hard and fast conclusions, nor should the reader expect any far-reaching syntheses. It will be enough if it can be established that there is indeed an intrinsic, if elusive, psychological connection between creativity and loss and that this connection lies at the heart of both the cancer stories and the clinical vignettes that take up the second half of the book. Beyond that, I would like to suggest that understanding this connection enables us, whether as professionals or as people personally connected to the dying, to respond better to the unique needs of the terminally ill individual. Put another way, if we can under- stand what it is that the naturally gifted, creative person brings to the situation of being a cancer sufferer, then we will be better able to understand how this same quality might be evoked from the outside through the mediation of a concerned other.

PSYCHOANALYTIC APPROACHES TO CREATIVITY

Freud was skeptical of psychoanalytic illumination of the nature of the artistic process. His works are liberally sprinkled with such declara- tions as "Where the artist gets his ability to create is no concern of psychology" (1913a, p. 187), and "Before the problem of the creative arts, analysis must, alas, lay down its arms" (1928, p. 177). Freud also thought that the end result of the artist's endeavor could not be judged psychoanalytically: "We have to admit that also the nature of artistic achievement is inaccessible to us psychoanalytically" (in Jones, 1957, p. 114). Freud's (1924b) judgments were consistently unequivocal: "It [psychoanalysis] can do nothing toward elucidating the nature of the artistic gift, nor can it explain the means by which the artist works—artistic technique" (p. 65).

What Freud did feel was possible was that psychoanalysis might shed some light on an artist's motives considered quite apart from any issues of talent or successful realization. For Freud, this more limited interpretive opportunity hinged on a rough equivalence between creative imaginings and the mechanisms of hysterical fantasy formation. In both, present perceptions are modified by way of fantasy to assimilate past emotional experiences; therein lies the possibility of interpreting the artist's motives from the circumstances of the artist's present and past life. The interpretive goal is already implicit in Freud's remarks in the Draft N manuscript sent to his friend Fliess in late May of 1897, which contains Freud's first known musings about the motives underlying creativity. By chance, the motive in Freud's example is a potentially fatal one:

> The mechanism of fiction is the same as that of hysterical fantasies. For his *Werther* Goethe combined something he had experienced, his love for Lotte Kastner, and something he had heard, the fate of young Jerusalem, who died by committing suicide. He was probably toying with the idea of killing himself and found a point of contact in that and identified himself with Jerusalem, to whom he lent a motive from his own love story. By means of this fantasy he protected himself from the consequences of his experience.
>
> So Shakespeare was right in juxtaposing fiction and madness (fine frenzy) [Masson, 1985, p. 251].

Freud (1908) further enlarged the scope of his inquiry to include the raw materials from which creative products are shaped:

> We laymen have always been intensely curious to know ... from what sources that strange being, the creative writer, draws his material and how he manages to make such an impression on us with it and to arouse in us emotions of which perhaps we had not even thought ourselves capable [p. 143].

Freud found the answer in daydreaming, the roots of which extended back to childhood:

Should we not look for the first traces of imaginative activity as early as in childhood? The child's best-loved and most intense occupation is with his play or games. Might we not say that every child at play behaves like a creative writer, in that he creates a world of his own, or, rather, re-arranges the things in his world in a new way which pleases him? It would be wrong to think he does not take that world seriously; on the contrary, he takes his play very seriously and he expends large amounts of emotion on it. The opposite of play is not what is serious but what is real. . . .

The creative writer does the same as the child at play. He creates a world of phantasy which he takes very seriously—that is, which he invests with large amounts of emotion—while separating it sharply from reality [p. 144]

It is from the last factor, the sharp demarcation from reality, that Freud goes on to derive art's curious ability to handle themes that in ordinary life are too painful to bear:

The unreality of the writer's imaginative world, however, has very important consequences for the technique of his art; for many things which, if they were real, could give no enjoyment, can do so in the play of phantasy, and many excitements which, in themselves, are actually distressing, can become a source of pleasure for the hearers and the spectators at the performance of a writer's work [p. 144].

Freud's observation is a typically shrewd one, but if we reflect on the previous chapters, its application to the cancer stories is less than clear cut. Certainly Michie's imagined bird of prey, Albino Falcon, exists in an imaginative, almost hallucinatory world sharply separated from reality. Therein lies at least 90% of its genius: in imagination it is safe to express the terrible rages that in reality would be insupportable. But what of Gitanjali's poems? And what of the strictly autobiographical nature of the cancer stories generally? They deal consistently with a painful reality, and they do so explicitly and intentionally. There is no imagined world here, at least not in the terms Freud speaks of, not in the terms of the usual fictive unrealities that underlie the special dispensations of the novelist.

To be sure, in the cancer stories something is clearly present by way of an imaginative distance, but it is hard to say exactly what that distance consists of. Certainly, it has nothing to do with imagining a sunny alternative to reality. None of our authors was occupied with fantasizing about a better place they might be, nor did they occupy us with any halcyon dispensations from the realities of a hospice bed. There is an imaginative distance, but it is brought to bear directly on a painful reality. Perhaps one can speak of an imagined inner space where present circumstances can be observed but where they do not intrude. But what does this tell us about creativity?

The English pediatrician and psychoanalyst D. W. Winnicott (1971) expanded on Freud's equation of play and creativity in ways that bear more directly on our topic. Winnicott described how between the fourth and sixth months of life, infants develop the capacity to create objects that they regard as substitutes for the real mother. Using a creative illusion, children are able to invest an inanimate object with life. Ordinarily, it is the child's first possession—thumb, blanket, teddy bear—which is so invested with the products of subjectivity. Investing that object with the content of its inner world, the child creates an illusion that allows it to stay in contact with its previous experiences of the protective mother. Winnicott called this invested object a "transitional object" because it signals the onset of a transition stage in which the child moves from a primary unity with the maternal environment to the development of a real self separate from the mother. The transitional object belongs neither to external reality nor to the internal world. It is both created by the infant and provided by the world outside the infant's subjectivity.

According to Winnicott, the transitional object and the various transitional phenomena that succeed it later in development form the foundation for all creative activity. Moreover, it is in this intermediate area between the external and internal worlds, where objects are both provided and at the same time invented, that cultural products derive their meaning generally. An audience at a theatrical performance, for example, invests the actors with a significance that, strictly speaking, they do not have. Yet that investment is crucial for the dramatic effect. It is only because the spectators can relate to the various roles on the basis of their own inner experiences that they can feel themselves moved along by the unfolding action called for by the script. The play is at once outside and inside.

An audience that did not do this, an audience that did not invest motives and feeling into the actors, in short a truly detached audience, would have an entirely different experience. That audience would see what is ordinarily not apparent in the theater, namely, that the action has all been foreordained by the playwright, that what will happen tonight is identical with what happened last night and will happen the same way tomorrow night. At best, such a detached audience could take only a certain mathematical interest in the evening, following the successive tableaus with a logician's pleasure in seeing various intricacies resolved. Indeed, just this sort of "theater of alienation," to use Brecht's term, is sometimes deliberately staged for political or ideological reasons, to thwart our ordinary emotional reactions and force us to see things in a new and sometimes chilling light.

Paradoxically, insofar as the transitional object is an actual object, something that endures in the external world and can be lost and rediscovered therein, it potentially represents the child's first meaningful experience of the "not-me." More precisely, it represents the child's first *acceptable* meaningful experience of the "not-me," of a "not-me" that nonetheless can be made "mine." As such, the transitional object represents both a foothold in reality and a guarantor of continuity; it becomes the talisman par excellence for warding off fear and anxiety. For the developing infant, still largely dependent on its mother for its basic feeling of self, the transitional object quickly comes to serve as the focus for organizing the first defenses against fears of losing her. It is also the basis for organizing the first defenses against depressive reactions based on the recognition that one has, at least for the moment, already lost her. The child who reaches to clutch its blanket as its mother leaves the room is a familiar enough sight, but, psychodynamically speaking, the phenomenon is a quite complicated one. In essence, the child is imagining something—the mother-child union—and is using that imagining to create something—its experience of the blanket—that will allow it both to tolerate its loss and to fashion a new experience for itself.

But depressive reactions in the child are not based on loss alone. They are also ushered in by a panoply of aggressive and destructive urges directed against the caretaking figure, urges that in their turn trigger concerns about having damaged the mother (psychoanalytically speaking, the maternal object) or otherwise having made her "bad." Our understanding of this class of mental phenomena stems principally from the work of Melanie Klein, whose hypotheses about infantile mentation have proved endlessly fruitful even if one rejects her highly metaphorical language and her unlikely datings in ascribing complex dynamics to newborns. Klein (1975) believed that the child enters into a "depressive position" and takes leave of an earlier "paranoid" position, when it recognizes that the mother is a whole person who can be hated as well as loved. The child thus comes to fear that its ambivalent feelings toward her, with their felt destructiveness and their accompaniment of real or fantasized attacks, might have damaged or destroyed her love for the child. As a result, the child feels guilt and, if this is not mediated by the mother's continuing availability, depressive despair.

Clearly, the ability to get into this position represents a developmental achievement for the infant. For Klein and her followers, the establishment of the depressive position goes hand and hand with the establishment of a reality-oriented ego. The intense feelings of loss that the child experiences as the result of its own attacks on the mother, whether fantasied or not, give rise to a wish to repair the lost, loved object and instill it with new life and wholeness (Segal, 1973). Though the ministrations of the actual mother continue to be crucial in mitigating depressive despair, the infant's success in working through this stage depends largely on its ability to restore the mother internally, for it is this fantasied internal object that is both the carrier of the felt goodness of the old narcissistic symbiosis and the principal recipient of the damages that infantile rage can inflict.

Hence, in a way unthinkable in the earlier paranoid stage, when the infant simply sought escape from persecutors, internal and external, real and imagined, in the depressive stage the child initiates reparative activities. These reparative activities, which are essential in the working through of the depressive position, and thus in the formation of the ego and the sense of reality, are animated throughout by the wish to restore, preserve, and recreate the lost happiness of symbiosis and so give the internal object external life. By the same token, these reparative activities also form the nuclei of the child's developing conscience or superego. It is because the child begins to feel that it is possible, through its own activity, to restore a preexisting and benign state of affairs that it first takes on the moral burden of ascribing badness to itself and seeking to make amends. The superego which commands this moral activity, in turn, partakes of the qualities of the good object.

These complex dynamics form the heart of the depressive stage, and their impact on the child is no less important than its fears of simple abandonment. And, just as the transitional object constitutes the child's first acceptable experience of the not-me and thus serves as a first defense against fears of loss, so too does it have a role to play in overcoming the special anxieties of the depressive stage. The teddy bear or blanket becomes the carrier of the infant's hopes that the good internal mother has not been destroyed, that her loving support can be recreated each time the infant feels threatened by the extent of its own anger. Though parents ordinarily do not pay attention to this side of things, the child's play with the transitional object can begin to take on frightful proportions as the object is successively annihilated and reinvented, with only a very gradual emergence of concern for the object's own "feelings" about all this. We do well here to bear in mind Freud's observations that play is "serious." It is indeed; for it is by playing that the small child first comes to terms with the potentially frightening world of its own passions.

And with the mention of play, we are reminded of our point of departure. If we accept Winnicott's (1971) logic that creativity first arises out of transitional phenomena, then there is reason to suppose that it does in fact have a special relation to themes of loss and mourning. Through play, the special form of its own creativity, the child first learns to be alone. Initially, the child plays "alone" in the presence of its mother and then later, with the introjection of the mother's supportive ego, it really plays alone. This is where ego strength, the capacity to be oneself by oneself, begins. Similarly, it is through creative, symbolic play that the child first learns to survive its own rages while keeping a sense of its basic goodness, and the goodness of its internal objects, intact. From the very beginning, it appears, creativity, loss, depression, mourning, and reparation are all intertwined.

THE THREAT OF MORTALITY

The special response of cancer authors or cancer artists is defined, first of all, by their preexisting capacities to create, capacities that seem to have broadened their ability to tolerate and to resolve threats to their psychic integrity. Artists and writers who are accustomed to creative activity have strengthened their sense of omnipotence and self-love; in the face of cancer, they can more readily respond to the experiences of deprivation, intense fear, and mourning without being overwhelmed by intense anger and hate. Writing the cancer book or painting the cancer picture is a powerful alternative to more primitive responses, such as denial and projective identification, by which, as we know from infancy, the ego might otherwise protect itself from despair. Despair threatens to overtake the ego only when the ego no longer has any faith in its ability to restore the good internal object.

The special response of the cancer author or artist is frequently apparent at the very first step in the psychooncological sequence, diagnosis. The fear of dying of cancer is often the fear of being overtaken by a bad internal object, symbolized by the tumor that is out to persecute and ultimately consume its victim. The race against this slow process of destruction can be successful only if the superego and the ego ideal, represented by the good internal object, can be recathected and the ego can still identify with them (Meerwein, 1989). The cancer sufferer who writes a book or creates a piece of art or offers a scientific contribution can justly hope to be recognized by the public and thereby satisfy omnipotent and narcissistic wishes, so badly damaged by the disease process, all with a gain of psychic pleasure and a diminution of fear. At the same time, he or she can thus counteract the malignant internal process symbolized by the cancerous tumor. Thereby, an identification with the superego and the ego ideal can yet be maintained. Thus, the cancer book or painting has a dual aspect: it represents a goodbye present, while at the same time it will endure after the artist's death and so ensure immortality. Then, end and endlessness seem identical, and the threatening reality is somehow suspended (Meerwein, 1989).

To understand the dual temporal aspect of the cancer book or painting, we should consider the concept of time from a developmental frame of reference. The newborn's preliminary experience of time begins with the disturbance of its bodily rhythms (Lichtenberg, 1983). The prototype for such an experience is hunger, the disturbance of comfortable satiation with consequent tension in the body. The infant who has previously experienced mother's satisfying its hunger can initially activate a hallucination of the "food-mother." With the child's growing experience that the mother usually does come in time to still its hunger, the ability for anticipation grows, and trust in the mother develops within the hunger-tension situation. We can say that this anticipation expresses a rudimentary time perspective, implying an incipient sense of a now, a before, and an afterward.

The infant who has to wait for the fulfillment of its wishes experiences the interval between the perception of hunger and its subsequent satisfaction as short or long. This represents the earliest experience of duration and, depending on the child's ability to anticipate satisfaction, the incipient perception of the various time sequences that are implicitly at stake (past, present, future) undergo substantial changes correspondingly. If the tension of waiting is tolerable, the child's affects during this period can be properly characterized as longings. As time progresses, however, and its hunger is still not satisfied, the child's affect changes and progresses into frustration and fear. Now the child grapples with the possibility that satisfaction might not come after all. Helplessness can set in, threatening the earlier sense of hope and trust, and the future turns into a dangerous time dimension. The younger the infant, the less is its ability to anticipate satisfaction in the face of mounting distress. Tension grows fast, and terror takes over. Fear turns into panic, and panic into powerlessness, rage, and hopelessness. The future is lost, and catastrophic anxiety becomes the only knowable present. In a traumatic situation, the child always experiences time as timelessness (Haefliger, 1988).

Timelessness can also have a positive aspect. When the infant is fully satisfied and satiated, it experiences a comfortable timelessness, an experience of eternity as an eternal present, where separation between present, past, and future is suspended, where there is no memory or wish, no anticipation, just an absorption in being. Freud, following his friend Romain Rolland, called this the "oceanic feeling." Describing the state in terms of the child's narcissistic balance, we would say that a high degree of fusion with the idealized internal object takes place. By contrast, the other potential aspect of timelessness, entailed in situations of deprivation and catastrophic anxiety, is exemplified by a sense of utter aloneness and closeness to the negative eternity of death. The opposite to the experience of the oceanic feeling is fragmentation: the world falls apart; all connections are destroyed.

At about the age of 12 months, the little child begins to understand the implication of the word soon. This understanding implies an incipient grasp of the concept of the future. Soon is not yet, not tomorrow, but "today." The concept of the past can be understood by the child around 36 months. It is at this age that the image of the good mother, who once satisfied the self, and the angry, bad aspects of the mother become fused together, initiating Klein's depressive position. In health, the secure integration of the opposites good self and bad self (within the child) and good object and bad object (within the image of the mother) becomes consolidated and generates the concepts of the real self and the real object. Emotional object constancy thus emerges at the same time as the child masters the concepts of the present, the past, and the future. True object constancy implies that the image of the real mother can survive the emotional vicissitudes, real and imagined, inherent in the parent–child relationship, but it also implies a sense of stability over time. Put another way, the real mother must be able to endure in the child's imagination across all three time dimensions, past, present, and future. The two processes, emotional integration and the mastery of time, go together at this age. This is also the developmental period when the superego is being formed, with its assimilation of parts of the idealized object into the ego ideal (Haefliger, 1988).

With the onset of cancer in the adult, the psychological structures governing both the concept of the self and the experience of the self and others in time face a massive threat that renders the ego ideal all the more important. If the cancer patient can identify with the timelessness of the ego ideal, then the bad internal objects are robbed of some of their destructive power. When I asked the painter and art educator Ruth Weissberg what had changed for her since her mastectomy three years earlier, she answered that it was her sense of time. She now experiences time as "a circle or a continuation, a river of humanity, where there are wounded and blessed ones and where there is regeneration." The content, as well as the form, of Weissberg's art illustrates this changed sense of time: her famous scroll painting, drawn on a big roll of paper, shows the circle of life with neither beginning nor end.

Doris Schwerin (1976) describes how she watched pigeons nesting on the ledge outside of her New York City apartment as she recovered psychologically from her mastectomy. Schwerin was first drawn just to observe them, then to help them to survive a cold winter, to raise nestlings, and to fight off marauders. In her mind, it was not only them she observed but herself and her own past: "I close in for a look at infancy again" (p. 28). She writes, "The two little pigeons and their parents had become my chances to connect with an ancient step, 'feeling' the nest, the past, the steps of transformation..." (p. 83). She describes how the first flight of the baby pigeon made her present time stand still, becoming "another still life, alive with time. Just time" (p. 99). The bird-watching connects her to her time of childhood and to her internal objects: "Where was Mama? Was she watching the first day I flew? Was she coming to feed me, beak to beak? How come Ma and Pa Smith [her names for the pigeon parents] 'knew' and she didn't" (p. 100). "Sunlight on the pigeon nursery ledge was pricking me with signals from my inner space," Schwerin adds (p. 109), describing her new connection to her internal world. She further observes, "past time unremembered and present time merge" (p. 113).

Watching the pigeons during a whole winter enabled Schwerin to get in touch with her own infancy and childhood; one can feel her working through the loss of her breast as she describes the pigeons guided by their strong parental instincts. The mourning, and the reintegration that followed, led in turn to both a stronger sense of self and an altered sense of time. Of a subsequent visit to the graves of her parents, Schwerin reflects on her lost breast and her changed body: "I am different and yet strangely whole, more whole than I've ever been" (p. 287). She wanted to say to her parents, "I took time in my hand and threw it up in the air" (p. 287). The multidimensional experience of watching the unfolding of nature's secrets, of being open to her own past secrets, and of writing about it enabled Schwerin to reintegrate time's different domains and to feel alive again.

The created product of the cancer writer is located between the patient's inner world and the reader's outer reality; it takes the form of a transitional object in an intermediate space of mourning. Weissberg's scroll painting and Schwerin's diary, like other art and literature created by cancer patients, provide transitional objects between outside and inside, between past time and present time, and allow for a temporary defense against an identification with timelessness in its traumatic, fragmenting aspect. That would be identical with psychic death, traumatic for the reader or viewer no less than for the patient.

What do cancer patients mourn? As we saw in Part I, the mourning at first is for the loss of the illusionary timelessness that we consider life to be, the sense of life security; only secondarily is the mourning for the loss of body parts and bodily functions, with their accustomed gratifications, and only at the very end is it for the ultimate sorrow, the loss of life itself. The mourning for life security can itself cause extremely painful longing. We could say it is a longing for the transitional phase, for the supportive, protective play space, and for the sense of time that is a part of that space. Cancer patients long for a creative defense with which they can approach their coming losses so they do not seem so overpowering.

As we discussed earlier, in the transitional phase of childhood creation through play helps the child to separate from the mother and to establish its own special relationship with reality. The discovery of a new form of literary or artistic endeavor in the guise of the cancer story or cancer painting, with its concomitant increase in the feeling of artistic omnipotence, helps artists with cancer to face separation, to mourn the losses, and to establish a relationship to the new realities they are forced to face. For many authors, the topic of cancer itself is sufficiently novel, and the challenges it presents sufficiently difficult, to constitute a major departure from their accustomed style of working. But, for others this is not enough, and it is not unusual to see an already successful artist take up an entirely new mode of expression. And, if the cancer should recur after an initial remission, it is also not unusual to see a second change in the mode of artistic expression. Many of the artists I interviewed responded in these ways. Ruth Reichstein, an anthropologist and violinist, abandoned her music and began to concentrate on poetry when her cancer was diagnosed. Then, when the cancer returned, she found that she could no longer write poetry; but she was moved to take up photography, and she occupied herself with taking pictures of trees, obsessed by the scars in the wood. When she was dying, these photographs inspired her to create her last poems. So spellbound was she by this inspiration that she was able to block out her intense pain, suspend the threatening reality of her impending death, and remain hopeful up until the very end. One of these poems is the following:

> Feder. Schlafend. Das Auge geschlossen.
> Fliegen! Ueber die Staedte, die Waelder, die Wiesen
> ueber die Wolken, die Winde, den Regen, den Tau.
> Der Sonne nah
> Unendlich der Raum
> Nie mehr stuerzen
> aus der Tiefe
> des Traums.

> Feather. Sleeping. The Eye closed.
> Flying! Over cities, woods, meadows,
> over clouds, winds, rain, dew,
> close to the sun.
> Infinite Space.

> Never again crash
> from the depth
> of the dream.
> —Reichstein (1990)

The establishment of new forms, whether through one's accustomed means of self-expression or through a novel kind of creative activity, tends to elicit pleasurable, satisfying feelings in spite of the life-threatening situation and helps repair the narcissistic damage brought about by the malignant process of cancer. The mourning engendered by the many losses entailed by cancer stimulates unconscious longings for the lost closeness with the primary object as well as a longing for a new gestalt and a new solution. As the transitional object in infancy could be used as a symbol for the absent mother, the cancer book, poem, or picture can become the mediating symbol of separation and togetherness, of dying and immortality.

The word "symbol" derives from the Greek word *symballein*, meaning to unite, to connect, to bring separate parts together. Symbols can reveal and communicate, as well as conceal. Symbols help artists to create order and aid in the development and definition of form. Symbolization through the creative process helps artists with cancer to organize their inner experience and to perceive their environment. For cancer patients it is particularly important to find a new gestalt for their overwhelming experiences and mold these experiences through the use of symbols, expressed in images. For Melanie Klein (1975), the ability to produce symbols is the basis of healthy ego development in childhood; similarly, the ability to create new symbols, even threatening ones, plays an important role in the creative response to a life-threatening illness.

We saw a number of these symbols in the first half of this book. For example, Diggelmann (1979), after he was confronted with the diagnosis of his brain tumor, took up his pen and wrote this passage:

> The doctors, who mean well, tell me day after day how strong the bad death flower grows in my head, grows roots, how it feels comfortable in the safety of the wall of my skull. It is blooming beautifully, the doctors tell me, and it is very connected to me as though it loved me. At night, I sit in front of the black window and hear in the quiet of my long road to death the begging voice of a new flower . . . [p. 22].

Like most of our cancer authors and artists, Diggelmann has open lines of communication between his psychic systems and thus easy access to primary-process thinking and imagery. Interestingly, during the creative process the artist's psychic functioning often appears devoid of repression. Diggelmann's imagery is typical in this regard: it addresses directly what one would otherwise ordinarily tend to suppress. Foregoing the usual comfort of not knowing, or at least of not paying attention, Diggelmann can use his symbol of the "death-flower" to bring order within himself. He creates a symbol that unites opposites within a new gestalt and a new form. The same is true for the following Janus-like symbol taken from Diggelmann's (1979) writing:

> . . . I am death and I am life. If you don't take me, death, in, don't expect me to appeal to you again as life. . . . I don't beg as death for your life. I give you your life as a gift in that I appear as death in front of you. Don't push me away, don't defend yourself. . . . You will eventually realize that it is not death who knocks on your window, but transformed life. [pp. 20-21].

Dying is a universal experience that has always found expression in art and literature and there it is usually colored by archetypal imagery spawned by the collective unconscious. Artists who are actually confronted with their own imminent death, however, must shape these universal images into very personal symbols answering to the artists' past experiences and to unconscious motives. The following poem on death by Claire Henze, a California-based photographer and writer, was created after her mastectomy and illustrates this well. Among other responses, Henze had tried to picture death for herself through a series of photographs, including one of a huge, unmanned motorcycle standing in the desert at Death Valley (Picture 1). Her poem amplifies that image:

To Death

Just a punk kid
who thinks he's hot shit
with your big bikes, guns, cameras,
power tools you don't even know how to use.
Get out of my house and quit following me!
I know you haven't come to raid my house.
It's me you're after.
With those black gloves that tease my throat.
But you can't make up your mind,
You just hang around in the shadows.
It's not so easy with me.
I won't fall down for you

or go down, or lie anywhere near you.
Tell him at least when my time comes
to send a man who has a way with women,
a man with continental flair
whose touch would make me forget the ache,
with whom I would go gladly
fitting my body to his.
In the meantime, punk shit bastard,
leave me alone. I'll take care of myself
                    —Henze (1987, p. 3).

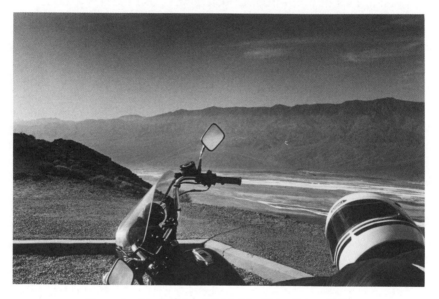

Picture 1.   *Death Valley*. Black/white. Claire Henze 1981.

Aggression and libido, frustration and gratification, all are essential for creative activity. Henze tries to unify these opposites in her image of death. This very particular symbol of death stems from Henze's unconscious and is fed by her early experiences. Death is here symbolized as an immature youth, not a man, yet one who threatens her and tries to seduce her at the same time. The artist aims to find a creative symbol for her life threat and her mourning by unifying opposites within one symbolic creation.

The unification of opposites is also very well illustrated in the following poem by Reichstein, the anthropologist turned poet:

Abwesend	*Absent*
Ein Glass Milch	A glass of milk
fand sich	I found
in deinem Zimmer	in your room
Die Milch	The milk
war fest	was firm
und Schimmel	and mildew
wuchs auf ihr	grew on it
wie Gras	like grass
auf einem frischen Grab	on a new grave

—Reichstein (1986, p. 27).

Reichstein, who wrote most of her published poems after the outbreak of her breast cancer, told me that writing these poems gave her the highest sense of happiness and satisfaction. She saw in them "a fusion of melody, form, and language" unreachable in any other art form. When artists with cancer create, they experience a great sense of fulfillment because an organic cohesiveness reconciling inside and outside can be accomplished. The artist's inside is no longer only an incubator for a malignant cancerous process, but is also the healthy soil for symbolization and form giving. The artist has the ability to give form to life and death and to creativity and mourning.

From a functional point of view, Michie's "Albino Falcon," or "A.F.," is a different kind of symbol altogether. Embodying the author's free floating anger, A.F. was stimulated into existence by the diagnosis of cancer and then sustained by its various complications such as radiation treatment. Through her strong, expressive symbol, Michie delegates her aggression and her will to take revenge to a protective entity outside herself. While she dutifully submits to a harsh treatment regimen, these impulses find satisfaction in the malicious adventures of this bird of prey, who is alive and active and vigilantly seeks out and attacks her foes. The self-healing function of this particular symbolization is clear: it allows the artist/patient to split off her aggression and project it onto her imagined avenger. From a psychological standpoint, technically speaking one could almost speak of projective identification here, as Michie both projects her anger and remains connected to it. But, by confining her aggression to her writing, Michie herself was able to stay calm and relaxed with her health care team. Moreover, grasping its psychic utility ought not distract us from recognizing the fact that A.F. also represents a creative achievement, one that might not have occurred to another patient. Like other cancer authors,

Michie discovered that, with the realization of cancer and its implications, she also developed an exceptional urge to symbolize and to create.

What all these strong symbolic expressions have in common is that they attempt to connect with someone or something in another realm. They seek to reach what is not directly reachable, to express in an imaginary realm that is not truly expressible, to traverse the boundary between the inside and the outside, between the world of the living and the world of the dying. Typically, the symbolic imagery tries to express the destructive process of cancer along with the restitutive and reparative processes that are part of art and literature.

Ruth Weissberg, the gifted painter and performance artist who was confronted with breast cancer a few years ago, in one of her subsequent performance pieces enacted the story of a swan who flies off to a distant place when it realizes that tumors are beginning to grow under its chest feathers. When it examines the tumors more carefully, however, they turn out to be little hummingbirds. Clearly, Weissberg's symbol of the hummingbird has a wishful aspect to it and contains the power of magic. But beyond that an important truth is contained in the image; for Weissberg the real tumor turned out to be a source of spirituality and creativity.

A similar image occurred to the German painter Richild Holt, and to much the same effect. After Holt had completed the last of her five mastectomy self-portraits, she suddenly rediscovered her heartbeat, which now felt "like a little bird in a cage" (cited in Tallmer, 1989, p. 4). Similarly, the bird also became an important symbol for the artist Hanna Wilke, who tamed a real bird that flew into her window three days after her mother died of breast cancer. She gave the bird her mother's Yiddish name, Chaya, from the Hebrew for "the living." When the bird was accidentally killed shortly after the mourning period for her mother was over, Wilke was given another bird, which kept her company and helped in her battle with the small nodular lymphoma that was diagnosed shortly afterward (Langer, 1989, p. 132).

For all three artists, birds, archetypal symbols for sublimation, imagination, and love, become the messengers from the world of the living to the world of the dying.

THE BODY RESTORED

Just as Aristotle argued that the sense of touch was primary, Winnicott (1958) and Melanie Klein (1975) have noted that for the infant the first reality is the reality of the body. That reality is tested through the infant's motor activity. Throughout our lives we express various symbolic connections between our bodies and the outside world. And within that imaginative landscape of the real—of the embodied—the hand has a special psychobiological significance and its own special history. From intrauterine life onward, the hand is closely allied to the mouth. In infancy, the hand carries oral tension from the mouth to the rest of the body(Hoffer, 1964). The writer's pen and the artist's brush are extensions of the hand and thus means of both expressing and purifying the body image in general. In a sense, the hand carries the tension of love and hate, of life and death, out onto the paper or canvas, just as in infancy the hand spreads stimulation from the mouth to the skin. When Matisse was asked how he could distinguish between his very good pictures and the lesser ones, he replied that he could feel the difference in his hand (Rose, 1980).

An artist's or writer's work is, first of all, always physical work, and creative art is one way of reexperiencing pleasurable bodily states. The heightened sensitivity that many artists have to their bodily sensations, as well as to perceptual reality, leads to an active search for a harmonious balance between bodily states and the forms of the external world. Psychological self-repair through writing and artistic expression always contains the unconscious wish that the finished product might reestablish the physical intactness that is being destroyed by the cancerous process. This is especially so for women who suffer from breast cancer, as we shall see in a later chapter. Israeli actress Nira Rabinowitz told me how she used the two days between the biopsy of her breast and the subsequent mastectomy to separate from her breast while memorializing it in photographs.

Ruth Reichstein, the Swiss poet, suffered from an inflammatory breast cancer that necessitated numerous skin transplants and found herself taking pictures of tree trunks, and especially of diseased and scarred bark. Only later did she realize that she had unconsciously found projected onto nature images of her own scars and her changing skin tissues. Even destructive changes in nature, she explained to me, slowly become an integrated part of that nature and eventually are experienced as aesthetically beautiful. Her choice of motifs for her photographs was one way to come to terms with her diseased skin and body. Her photographs and her poems alike can be understood as a self-healing attempt to come to terms with her physical scars; she hoped to be able to reintegrate her scars into her body image, as nature is able to accept its defects as part of a natural process and uses them to reestablish physical integrity.

The writer and photographer Henze, in the initial period after the mastectomy, took black and white photographs of her two little children naked. These snapshots were done with a cheap, plastic camera, and the images were foggy and out of focus, mirroring the artist's own blurred perception during the period immediately following her diagnosis. Today Henze realizes that acting on the urge to capture her children's strong, healthy, intact bodies on film helped her to balance her feelings toward her own body, which had been mutilated through mastectomy. The creative act helped her to maintain a sense of psychological intactness and wholeness, thus preparing her to heal the narcissistic wound.

Similarly, the German painter Richild Holt painted herself naked and whole as she was confronted with a very bleak prognosis of her malignant breast cancer. As she describes it, on hearing the news she went utterly

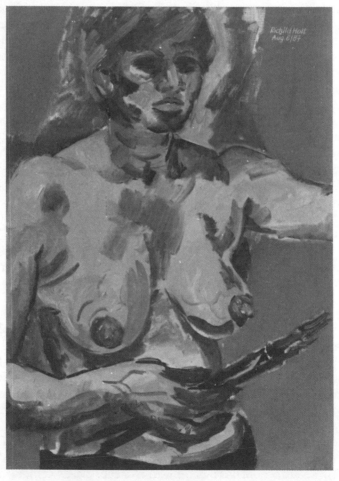

Picture 2. *Death Sentence, August 6, 1987.* Oil on canvas, 50 × 70 in.
Richild Holt.

to pieces, but she was still able to paint for three hours straight and afterward felt calmer. Though her painting, entitled "Death Sentence," (Picture 2) shows her still physically intact, it reveals her profound distress in the lack of articulation and heavy shading of her face. Three days later, after a second medical examination, where the death verdict was somewhat revised, Holt again painted herself with two breasts; but this time her face, with her angled glance directed at the viewer, is clearly visible above. (Picture 3) Following her mastectomy, the day her bandages came off she was in great pain; but with the protection of a nurse, Holt managed to paint

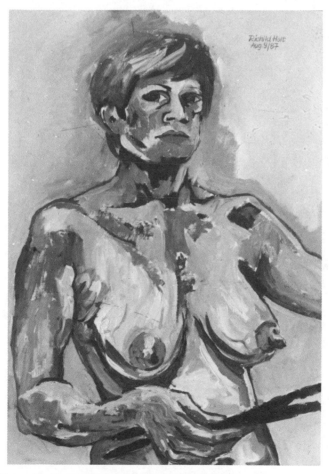

Picture 3. *Revised Sentence, August 9, 1987.* Oil on canvas, 50 × 70 in.
Richild Holt.

a third self-portrait while still in her hospital room (Picture 4). Again, she felt calmer afterward. In this painting the painter's injured chest is depicted clearly and without sentiment . . . her glance is head-on and direct.

The last two of Holt's self-portraits, as she explained to me in a letter, were created in an attempt to get to know the empty space on her chest better and to familiarize herself with this new, mutilated body: "I had to paint these 'cancer pictures' to comprehend what actually happened." In the first of this final pair there seems to be a revisitation of the death-fear, in the form of shading about the face (Picture 5), but in the second, there

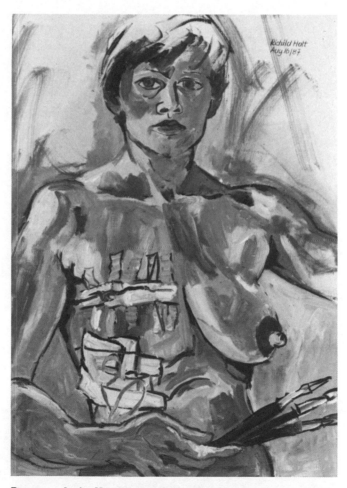

Picture 4. *In the Hospital, August 16, 1987.* Oil on canvas, 50 × 70 in.
Richild Holt.

now appears an integration of all the elements of the previous paintings, and the artist's hand moves protectively to cover her wounds (Picture 6). The gesture reflects hope, and indeed it was at this point that Holt rediscovered her heart fluttering "like a little bird in a cage." The act of painting had facilitated both an integration of the new body-self and the acceptance of a new life-gestalt with which Holt could identify. From an artistic standpoint, Holt believes that one goal of the artist is to force into the foreground a heightened sense of awareness of oneself and one's body and that in illness this awareness must be able to both confront and contain the painful truth. She also believes, and I think this is true for all people who are confronted with cancer, that in its raw, unformed, and unexpressed state the bodily truth of disease is extremely painful psychologically and almost unbearable.

Deena Metzger, a feminist writer and poet, actually tattooed around her chest scar a growing tree. The following poem, written shortly thereafter, illustrates her powerful need for transformation and her drive to give form to her experience, using her imagination as the major force of healing:

> *I Am No Longer Afraid*
>
> I am no longer afraid of mirrors where I see the sign
>   of the Amazon, the one who shoots arrows.
> There was a fine red line across my chest where a
>   knife entered, but now
> a branch winds about the scar and travels from arm
>   to heart.
> Green leaves cover the branch, grapes hang there
>   and a bird appears.
> What grows in me now is vital and does not cause
>   me harm. I think the bird is singing.
> I have relinquished some of the scars.
> I have designed my chest with the care given to an
>   illuminated manuscript.
> I am no longer ashamed to make love. Love is a
>   battle I can win.
> I have the body of a warrior who does not kill or
>   wound.
> On the book of my body, I have permanently
>   inscribed a tree
>   —Metzger (1983, p. 194)

This poem, like her other works from this period, illustrates how Metzger enlisted her creative power to feel whole and intact again.

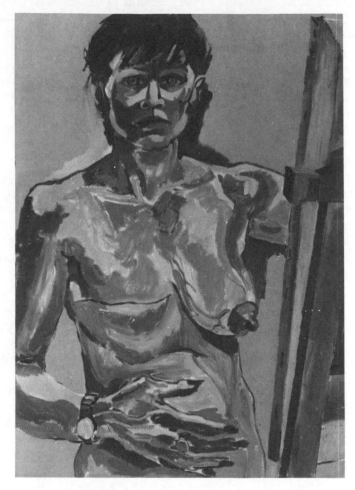

Picture 5. *September 1, 1987*. Oil on canvas, 50 × 70 in. Richild Holt.

The sculptor Nancy Fried uses her own changed chest as the basis for much of her work. Her headless torsos in bronze and terra cotta, which focus on her chest with its single heavy breast and its horizontal mastectomy scar, reveal an acceptance of her new, changed body. "I had to do it to heal myself," Fried says. The beautifully integrated pieces that she has executed since then reveal an aesthetic completeness and demonstrate her successful attempt at self-healing. The sculpting allowed for the discovery of a new gestalt and an acceptance of a new, changed body (Pictures 7 and 8).

Women, perhaps more than men, need to come to terms with the changes in their bodies. From puberty to pregnancy to postmenopause,

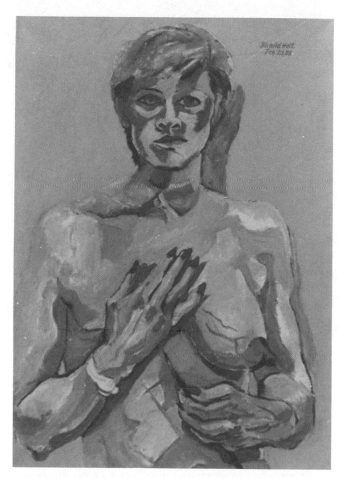

Picture 6. *February 1988*. Oil on canvas, 50 × 70 in. Richild Holt.

with their associated possibilities of a flat chest or scarred belly, bodily transformations are facts of a woman's physical evolution. If this normal evolution is changed or speeded up through the malignant processes of cancer, then the need to hold on to an image of the intact, healthy body becomes all the more important and constitutes one of the major wishes of the artist. Thus, Rabinowitz and Holt memorized, and memorialized, their still intact breasts by photographing or painting them in the days before their mastectomies. Similarly in an unconscious way, Henze was moved to photograph the healthy bodies of her children, including the still immature, flat, but pure chest of her little girl.

By the same token, women often appear more ready to deal directly

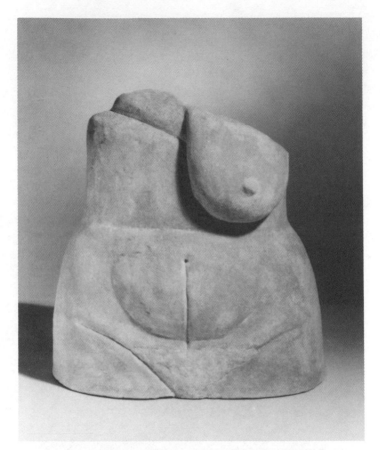

Picture 7.   *Torso*. Terra cotta, 10 × 10 ½ × 9 in. Nancy Fried 1987.
Photographed by Allan Finkleman Studio, New York City.

with the physical changes brought on by cancer and by surgery; perhaps direct artistic expression is more tolerable for a woman than it is for a man, whose physical changes are part of a much slower aging process. The woman patient takes her body as a frame of reference even when the cancer does not affect an emotionally laden organ like the breast. Recall the image used by the writer Maya Beutler (1980) as she described the feeling of trying, with her mouth still anaesthetized from her neck operation, to utter her first sounds: "Suddenly I am a woman, I push and press, tiny pieces of wet life can shoot out, if I just continue pushing" (p. 79).

FORMAL ASPECTS

Whether through painting, photography, performances, or writing, the artist seeks to form and transform the physical experience of cancer into

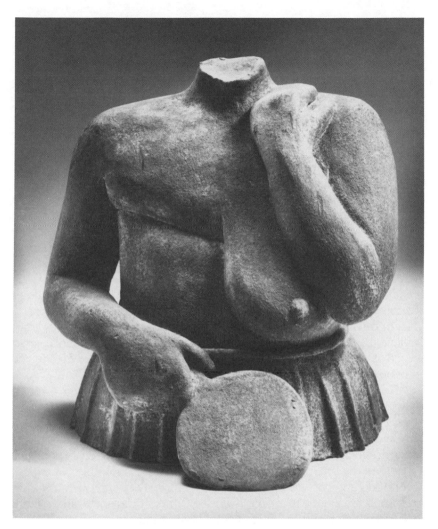

Picture 8. *The Hand Mirror.* Terra cotta, 10 × 10 ½ × 9 in. Nancy Fried 1987.
Photographed by Allan Finkleman Studio, New York City.

a completely new gestalt. An important aspect of this process is the use of form as a means of unifying the experience. Form becomes not only the carrier of unconscious wishes to regain the intact body, but also the means for shaping the rediscovered creative self, that part of the artist that is still alive and growing. Form becomes, as well, the carrier of another great wish, to reestablish a primary narcissistic balance undisturbed by threats of separation. In the unity of a literary or artistic form, and not only in the harmonious being-with-oneself of the creative process, the creative artist can search unconsciously for the original unity of mother and child. The structural coherence of a literary form can help overcome the painful separation of subject and object; likewise, it can temporarily suspend the passing of time, creating a new sense of a pleasurable duration where past and future are combined in the fullness of the present.

In fashioning the unity of a successfully executed work, the writer's ego secures a sense of omnipotence and self-love; from a psychodynamic perspective, the artist or writer inwardly enjoys the love of the mother once again, thereby overcoming the trauma of separation. Ordinary experience, and most especially the ordinary experience of a hospital bed, is broken up into disconnected pieces. Creative experience, by contrast, carries within itself its own wholeness and continuity.

Literary and artistic forms define the boundaries that govern the relations of, and conflicts between, wish and reality, objective circumstance and subjective fantasy. Form mediates between what is held to be inside and what outside and thus gives definition to the experience. In one sense, literary content is but a subjective moment contained and established by the objectifying form. In this respect, the content of each literary work is already largely given once the form has been selected. Freud, in his studies of Leonardo da Vinci (1910) and Michelangelo (1914), showed that aspects of form can reveal to us something about the psychology of the artist. Susanne Langer (1953), whose ideas developed out of symbolic logic, arrived at the proposition, that form is a direct expression of feeling and emotion.

From a psychological standpoint, the ability of a chosen form to organize the expression of uncontrolled fantasies and to link these fantasies to reality enables the writer to work productively within his subjective situation. In this context, form becomes the principle of selectivity governing between fantasy and reality, between drives and the reality principle; it mediates the artist's choices with regard to the dichotomies of experience: inside and outside, wish and reality, subjectivity and objectivity. By structuring fantasy in this way, form yields an intermediate area where social acceptance and social integration persist unchanged.

Form also tells us about the structure of the artist/patient's ego. It assists in the functions of defense, drive neutralization, reality testing, and selective drive discharge. The pleasure of form derives not only from the discharge of those drive impulses which it selectively allows expression, but also from the defenses against those drives, defenses that acquire a gracefulness through their integration into the overall formal structure of the work. Take, for example, the deceptively simple literary form of Michie's lists, described in Part I. Upon hearing the news that she has cancer, the author consoles herself by writing down a list of things she no longer has to do, such as wash delicate things by hand or give large dinner parties or learn the metric system. It is a catalogue of life's nuisances, a reminder that we are not always so pleased with our corporeal existence and that, indeed, there are some things in it that we would readily give up. At first glance, the matter seems to speak for itself. But there is an important formal element involved here. The loose structure of the list facilitates the use of humor as a defense, since it allows the odd and irreverent thought free play while making its own contribution to the force of the content. For the suggestion, carried artistically by the fact that it is a list, is that all these things must be written down lest they be forgotten. That is why we usually make lists, to keep from forgetting things—as though it were possible to forget what was really at stake here. Thus does Michie keep herself, and her reader, from being overwhelmed by the threatening news of her cancer, the one thing that it would be virtually impossible to forget.

Webster's poem, "Bulletins From a War," whose strict, terse form is in keeping with the title, conveys an entirely different feeling and betrays an entirely different psychic organization. The form, suitable for a war-room dispatch, facilitates the aggressive content, with its images of an armed struggle and an uncertain truce. And just as the poet feels attacked by her cancer, her poetic style allows her to counterattack in her turn, her rage and her bitterness being all the more freely expressed because they are well contained by the form and thus will not hurt anybody. Form melds into content and content merges back into form:

Bulletins From a War

Civil war. My body is
the battleground.
Left breast falls first.
One lumpy legion conceals
treacherous intent.
Occupied territory:
The lymph system.
Suspected of abetting
the enemy,
ovaries are sacrificed.
Five-year cease fire
follows...
                    —Webster (1980, p. 35)

By contrast, though they are almost equally succinct, the form of most of Gitanjali's poems maintains a sense of balance and proportion; like the content of her work, Gitanjali's use of form, with its consistently contemplative beauty, is put in the service of superego goals. The form no less than the content works to provide an inner, structural security wherein her values endure unchanged. Her feelings can be observed, and honored, but they are not allowed to break the bounds of her even, always temperate verse. The writer who withdraws in this way behind the aesthetic safety of form both flees and accepts reality. At a distance from reality, but yet in contact with it, Gitanjali can analyze her situation and is thus enabled either to contain her feelings or to act on them as she pleases. The dramatic impact of her poems on the reader depends in part on the fact that in the end she does neither: her contemplation remains eternally balanced at the moment of decision, when both action and suppression are of equal weight.

The poignant inner contradictions of works like Gitanjali's ultimately grow out of the ambiguous relation of literature to society in general. Writers write both for their own satisfaction, and for an audience. The written word thus potentially resocializes the writer, while at the same time it allows the writer to remain alone. In Gitanjali's case this double function was enacted by the teenager herself. She at once hid the poems, so as not to upset her mother, even as she saved them from destruction, so that they would endure. While creating them she could cling to the comfort of knowing that they would be found after her death, a thought that must have eased her sense of emotional isolation and her fear of dying.

The same ambiguity in terms of society regularly attends the keeping of diaries, logs, and journals, and the work of cancer patients is no different in this regard. The relative privacy inherent in a journal or a diary constitutes a provisional promise that its contents might yet be kept secret. That in itself implies a sense of restraint, one that can be enlisted to buttress other formal devices meant to realize superego goals. For example, in the following excerpt from the diary of Dora Hauri (1982), the author begins with the tersest imaginable form, entirely in keeping with her austere sensibility generally. But in short order her guilt begins to get loose, stretching the frame; and then it threatens to turn into a remembered rage, one that can be contained only by a further symbolization that goes well beyond the bounds of her heretofore conventional discourse. And yet the whole of Hauri's statement is still constrained, and the superego demands satisfied, partially by virtue of its being, in the end, not a public outburst but an altogether discreet entry in a diary:

> November 16th, 1978
>> Knot in the breast.
>> No period.
>> Tiredness.
>> What was it? The smoking? The drinking? The addiction
> to movement. My rearing up in protest? A spurt of flame [p. 9].

The tighter and more rigid the artistic structure becomes, the more distant the author is from libidinal satisfaction, from the pleasurable sensations of the still living body and the satisfactions it can find in closeness to desire's objects. The payoff for the artist's or writer's inner mental economy lies in heightened feelings of self-control and mastery and the pride and self-satisfaction that such control can bring. But, at the extreme, the endeavor can reach grandiose proportions. Here artistic activity can become rigidly defensive; in such cases we can speak of what Hagglund (1978) has described as phallic creativity. Phallic creativity ensues when, from a psychological standpoint, the artist attempts to condense with castration anxiety issues arising out of separation, and then to abolish both by reaffirming the intactness and productivity of the self. In such instances, the act of creating becomes an entirely narcissistic experience in which the artist indulges the desire to be big, strong, admired, and so on, and whatever talent he might possess is used to build the sense of self ever higher. It is the artistic equivalent of the familiar proclamation, "I never felt better," though given that self-involvement can be expressed equally well in negative terms, it can also take the form of "Look what I have dealt with; look what I have overcome." When such a defense occurs in a cancer writer or painter, the attempt will be made to deny the inner emotional resonances of the circumstances: the writer is no longer alone, has not been abandoned, is not worthless, and so forth. Often enough, this kind of response enables the cancer sufferer to persevere in his or her artistic activity right up to the moment of death; it does not, however, eliminate separation anxiety, nor does it allow a working through of the issues. As a result, at the end there is only cessation, not acceptance.

Hagglund's (1978) description of phallic creativity is conceptually quite close to what Melanie Klein termed the "manic defense." According to Klein and her followers, the manic defense is characterized by a denial of psychic reality, a sense of omnipotent control and command, and a partial regression to the paranoid position with a resurgence in the archaic defenses of splitting, primitive idealization, denial, and projective identification (Segal, 1973). The aim of manic reparation is to repair the object in such a way that loss and guilt are never really experienced. From a psychodynamic perspective, it is as though the good aspects of the object have been taken into the self and made subject to the individual's control, so that not only is the whole infantile drama of anger, grief, and reparation supervened, but the very fact of separateness is denied as well. That is why phallic creativity is not an extension or transformation of mourning so much as a defense against it. There is no experience of grief, for it is precisely this emotion that has been circumvented, its place being taken by a sense of triumph and heightened self-esteem. Not until the phallic defense has sufficiently subsided can actual creativity be attained which will help the patient work through the necessary mourning (Hagglund, 1978).

In my review of the cancer literature, I have chosen to explore only one phallically creative book, *Mars*, by the Swiss writer Fritz Zorn (1977), which I discuss later. However, I did find several such books. Many of them are factual diaries from which all the personal feelings and fantasies of the authors have been systematically excluded in favor of polemical material, such as attacks on the medical establishment, grievances against family members or specific physicians, and proposals for different kinds of alternative treatment methods. Then there are those books in which religion is primarily used not as a consolation, nor as a means of contemplating ultimate meanings, but as a defense against facing disappointment and anger.

A good example of the latter is in Mary Higginbotham's *With Each Passing Moment* (1974). Higginbotham describes how, following her operation for cancer of the colon, an extremely humiliating and painful medical procedure, had to be repeated because the first doctor had inserted the wrong tube. Higginbotham's initial plaint is human and readily understandable: "Now it would be necessary to go through all of that again. How could I stand it?" (p. 15). But no sooner is that thought out than it is immediately superceded by another, which leans heavily on Corinthians 4:17, "Why should my heart complain, when wisdom, truth, and love direct the stroke, inflict the pain, and point to joys above" (p. 15). And even this is not enough, as Higginbotham goes on to say "How ashamed I felt by my unvoiced complaining. Unvoiced, yes, but God knew. Had not my God said, 'I am with you always' (Matthew 28:20)" (p. 15). What books such as Higginbotham's typically have in common is a refusal by their authors to come to grips with fear, loss, and mourning. Owing to their strongly defensive character, their formal and artistic values are very limited. So, too, revealingly, is their ability to console.

SHARED REPARATION

With the mention of consolation, we come to a final consideration in regard to the cancer stories: their ability to move us in ways we would not have imagined possible. As all who have found themselves touched by the authors of the first half of this book are aware, the cancer story or the cancer poem not only reflects its creator, but communicates to the reader as well. Its content and form convey the writer's inner reality to the reader, making emotional satisfaction possible within the reality principle. Just as we view the child's play from both inside and outside, so too do we view the artist's expression from both perspectives at once. As adults, we readily feel the emotions the child invests in play. In similar fashion, when we read a story or poem or view a picture, we can experience the emotions that the artist has invested in his or her creation. The creative product is located in the space between spectator or audience and the artist. It is a transitional object, a bridge between the inner and outer worlds, which both artist and audience can cross together. In this borderland of experience, the barrier between self and object is eliminated as the two become dialectically united, reciprocal terms that imply one another.

As for the recipient's sense of having been uplifted, Segal (1952), taking a term from Freud's analysis of the pleasure of wit, suggests that the public is "bribed" into aesthetic pleasure through "an identification of ourselves with the work of art as a whole and the whole internal world of the artist as represented by his work" (p. 204). She describes this as an unconscious reliving of the artist's experience of creation, constituting from a conceptual point of view an unconscious identification. Through that unconscious identification with the act of creating, we encounter again our own early depressive anxieties and once more experience the successful mourning that enables us to reestablish our own internal objects and our own internal world. The result of reliving these experiences unconsciously as we negotiate the aesthetic journey constituted by a work of art is a feeling of being reintegrated and enriched (Segal, 1952).

The experience of integration and enrichment is not any less true when the subject matter addressed by the act of creation is mortality. To be sure, when we are moved deeply by a cancer story, it is in part because the work embodies a profound, deep experience of the juncture of life with death with which we can identify. Not only does this archetypal imagery of death and loss surface in visible manifestations in these stories, resonating with the reader's collective unconscious, but the cancer artists symbolically express highly individual and personal experiences, which cannot help but intrigue us even as we approach them ever so cautiously. But to be truly consoling, the cancer story must go beyond its theme; it must contain within itself the creative adventure inherent in any successful work of art or literature and demonstrate that the adventure retains its essential goodness despite the topic. Then, as readers or spectators, we can unconsciously relive the artist's personal experience of loss and mourning and can share in the artist's sense of transformation and symbolic realization. The artist's or writer's disciplined observance of a form, meanwhile, provides a protective sense of detachment and keeps us, no less than the creator, from being emotionally overwhelmed. As readers or spectators, we can thus identify with the artist's enduring sense of wholeness and goodness and share in the unconscious communion with the good internal object as it is expressed in the work.

10

BREAST CANCER—
WRITING AS
PSYCHOLOGICAL SELF-REPAIR

With the help of literary examples taken from 10 books written by women during or after the acute phase of breast cancer, and with two clinical case vignettes, this chapter illustrates different ways of dealing with the losses accompanying breast cancer and attempts to show how the content of the cancer book or poem expresses different aspects of the mourning process as well as how the book or the poem itself can take the form of a new object, a healthy, life-giving breast. Writing the cancer book, which is often experienced as an inner necessity, allows the author to use creativity as a way of channeling the aggressive impulses engendered by her identification with the aggressive, malignant process of the illness and its accompanying unconscious fantasy of a destructive invasion of bad inner objects. Thus equilibrium within the ego is restored and the depressive reaction is relieved. By writing and publishing her book, the author is able to transform the very private experience of loss and mourning into a more universal one. By sharing this experience with the reader, she is able to accept her closeness to death and rebuild her badly damaged narcissistic integrity. Psychological self-repair through writing and creating following a mastectomy can be successful only if the threat of death and the loss of the breast are counterbalanced by love of life and by an identification with the good internal object—the good breast. Then new life, in the form of an artistic creation, can be born.

Ordinarily, mourning is a normal self-limiting process. Freud (1917) writes:

> Mourning is regularly the reaction to the loss of a loved person , or to the loss of some abstraction which has taken the

place of one, such as one's country, liberty, an idea, and so on.
. . . Although mourning involves grave departures from the
normal attitude to life, it never occurs to us to regard it as a
pathological condition. . . . We rely on its being overcome after
a certain lapse of time. . . . [pp. 243–244].

Freud goes on to say that profound mourning induces a lack of interest in
the outside world, which becomes impoverished and empty, and a turning
away from activities that are not connected to the lost object. As the
grieving person turns away from reality, reactions closely associated with
depression (melancholia) develop. These include the loss of the capacity
to love, self-reproach, and a loss of self-respect owing to the emptying of
the ego.

Every woman who loses her breast, regardless of her age and marital
status, has a depressive reaction, even though she might initially repress or
deny it. Often a feeling of great helplessness develops a few weeks after
the actual loss of the breast and reflects an increasing realization of the
implications of the diagnosis of cancer. Realizing that she will never be
able to restore her physical completeness nor deny the reality of death,
after the initial adaptive denial, the patient can fall into a state of utter
hopelessness and resignation In reaction to the loss of her ideal past, she
may capitulate and retreat. The capitulation often goes hand in hand with
a generalized inhibition of drives and ego functions. The patient then
becomes depressed in the classical sense.

Another reaction that can follow the initial normal depressive reaction is personal protest, a wish to fight the discontent, resentment, and fear
and to search for different, more active ways of dealing with the great loss
of the beautiful and highly libidinal organ that is filled with multiple
symbolic meanings. This internal rebellion leads to abandonment of the
pursuit of the ideal state of being a healthy woman with two breasts and
initiates active mourning work. The void that developed as a result of the
loss of the breast can then be filled with new ideas and, reflecting a wish
to change and attack old life-styles, a creative breakdown of old perceptions and images. The urge to change and break old habits, however,
needs to be balanced by a strong urge to rebuild and recombine old
elements and emotions into something new and satisfying. This inner
process of rebellion and change is very difficult to manage, especially for
a woman who has just lost a breast since she is frequently also confronted
with premature menopause due to chemotherapy or hysterectomy. She
fears that the change of her body will not only sap her physical energy and
deprive her of procreativity but will also take away her creativity.

The very act of writing a book about one's experience with breast
cancer initiates a mourning process. It is an active attempt to overcome-

one's depressive and destructive inclinations by transforming the threatening experience into a creative, constructive activity that can be shared with other women and men. If the book or poem contains a balanced interplay between pretense, fantasy, and the acceptance of a new reality, the writer can, together with the reader, mourn her lost breast and her lost sense of infinite life. Her cancer book then embodies a new vitality and at the same time serves as a memorial to the loss and working through process, an act of reparation with which the reader can identify. The writer gives to the reader the present of an intense, new, and valuable experience of dealing with the threat and the loss in a palpable form; in the giving, the writer also helps rebuild her own badly damaged narcissistic self. Lorde (1980) describes the following:

> I am writing this now in a new year, recalling, trying to piece together that chunk of my recent past, so that I or anyone else in need or desire, can dip into it at will if necessary to find the ingredients with which to build a wider construct. . . . I am also writing to sort out for myself who I was and was becoming throughout that time. . . .
> I am writing across a gap so filled with death—real death ... that it is hard to believe that I am still so very much alive and writing this [p. 53].

Lorde writes of learning "to transform silence into language and action... learning to put fear into perspective" (p. 20). Her experience of breast cancer thus acquires value as she tries "to give it a voice, to share it for use, that the pain not be wasted" (p. 16).

LOSSES WHEN FACED WITH BREAST CANCER

What are the losses that women with breast cancer experience? The following words by Hauri (1982) describe the many losses she suffered in her short fight with terminal breast cancer:

> With my disease and my being ill I lose my security and feelings of superiority, shyness and shame suddenly overcome me. I can no longer deal with my illness. . . . Till I die I will observe all the things which were taken from me: health, beauty, security, physical strength, confidence, profession, lust for life, independence. Naked, bare and exposed I will lie there in the end [p. 63].

This statement by a patient whose breast cancer turned out to be terminal typifies the losses experienced by most women who have breast cancer.

Christine Lenker (1984) describes the reaction she had after her doctor told her that she had cancer:

> I felt total hopelessness. Past and future were turned off; there was no despair, just a dumb emptiness, loneliness. I Left the doctor's office as though in a trance. I went to the car. I sat behind the wheel. I caught myself thinking: "I hope I don't cause an accident in my state". And then this thought seemed totally irrelevant, since I was now faced with something that seemed so much worse [pp. 14–15].

The patient's first loss after diagnosis is the loss of the fantasy of immortality that we all harbor deep down in our unconscious. Freud (1915) accurately described the experience when he wrote:

> We were, of course, prepared to maintain that death was the necessary outcome of life. . . . In reality, however, we were accustomed to behave as if it were otherwise. We showed an unmistakable tendency to put death to one side, to eliminate it from life. We tried to hush it up. . . . That is as though it were our own death, of course. . . . It is indeed impossible to imagine one's own death. . . . In the unconscious every one of us is convinced of his own immortality [p. 289].

After the shock of this first loss—this initial loss of the world—is over, the loss of the breast follows. All the literary quotations in this chapter are from women who underwent radical or modified mastectomies, which means that the entire breast, not only the tumor, was surgically removed. For every woman this is a severe narcissistic trauma. Betty Rollin (1976) describes the evening before her mastectomy:

> Without taking my eyes off the breast in the mirror, I put my hand over the left one, the one with the lump. I flattened the breast as much as I could, trying to imagine what it would look like if it weren't there. I wondered if they would scoop it out like a melon ball, and whether there'd be a hole. I took my hand away and looked at the breast the way it was. I looked at it as if it were a person I loved whom I would not see again. My throat swelled and my eyes filled up. I pulled my nightgown off the hook and over my head, fumbled in the medicine chest for

another Valium, found it, swallowed it, blew my nose, got into bed, and then it was Sunday [p. 52].

After her mastectomy, Hauri (1982) describes the trauma in her diary:

June 4th, 1979
I can't be consoled. I am badly mutilated, I hate people, the feeling of dying away.
Honky Tonk Woman
Honky Tonk Girl.
How I feel when I look at my breast. Alone I look in the mirror, I look at myself, what has become of me. No, it is not vanity.

May 29th, 1979
I am not beautiful anymore; it was beautiful to be beautiful. Who will see me crying, who will see this sadness?   [pp. 21-22].

The sight of the empty part of her chest makes Hauri, a divorced woman involved in a relationship with a man, feel suddenly alone. The loss of her beauty, in addition to the loss of her breast, intensifies her feeling of abandonment.

Reimann (1984) writes in her diary after her mastectomy:

December 25th, 1968
Annoyed and anxious, because my arm hurts.... Half a human being, bisected woman, halved woman. The horrors when waking up in the morning. I dream each night of dismemberment, and in the evening when I undress this feeling of strangeness: I look without horror at my scar. This can't be me; this cannot have happened to me. But it did [p. 291].

The dominant loss for Reimann, when she looks at her one-breasted chest, is of her identity: "This feeling of strangeness. This can't be me. This cannot have happened to me. But it did." In writing, she tries to fight against the strong need for denial she feels throughout the entire course of her malignant disease. Sometimes the denial becomes so strong that she totally loses her sustaining sense of identity as a successful writer and becomes clinically depressed. With professional help and a more open doctor–patient relationship, she subsequently regained self-confidence and was able to fight her fear and mourn her losses through writing.

Maxi Wander (1980), married, mother of one son (she lost a daughter in an accident), expresses the sudden loss of her youth following her mastectomy:

November 15th
   Other women age slowly, barely recognizing it. I aged in one Fall, a cut body which will never attract a man again. I will never be able to undress without shame on the beach. The body I loved is put out of commission for ever. I can't believe it, it is too horrible [p. 72].

With the following poem, Claire Henze (1987), the writer and photographer, mourns the mothering aspects of her breast. Although she can no longer nourish beautiful babies, she can create beautiful poems:

To My Daughter

You have the breasts now
Your baby nipple buds
will bloom one day
a discovery of roses
Cherish them
as you would your very inmost self.
Let them and you
be free of these cells
that can't stop growing,
that are fed by female blood.
May you grow beautiful babies
and beautiful breasts.
You will never remember
how you kissed the scar,
just like a scraped knee,
to make it better,
But I will.
You will never remember
how I looked with two breasts.
You are only two years old.
But I will
                    —Henze (1987, p. 48)

The more sexual, sensual aspects of her loss, Henze mourns in the following poem, which is dedicated to her son:

To My Son

Perhaps because of me
you will be a man to whom
breasts are not just boobs, knockers, jugs, tits
and calendar art.
Perhaps you will know
that any part of the body
is as worthy as another,
that there is beauty in
asymmetry,
that a breast only covers
the heart underneath,
that skin is the most erogenous organ,
that women are strong,
that men may weep
and that only lizards
grow new tails
                    —Henze (1987, p. 48)

The emphasis in the previous quotations was on the loss of the breast. In the following statements, the women focus less on the lost breast than on the breast that remains. At the time of mastectomy, Rollin (1976) was married but without children. She compares her healthy breast, saved from destruction, to a healthy baby:

> On the left half of my chest, where a breast had been, was a flat, lumpy surface like the ground, covered with, instead of dirt, skin. Across the surface, a long, horizontal, red, puffy welt meandered crazily from the center of my chest, where a cleavage once was, to the other side, under the arm, and around toward the back. And alongside this little Hiroshima of the torso, on the unbombed half, grotesque by contrast, lay a right breast, pretty and whole as a healthy baby [p. 146].

Lorde (1980), who describes herself as a "black, lesbian poet," writes clearly about her need to accept her one-breasted body while mourning the breast she lost:

> I looked at the large gentle curve my left breast made under the pajama top, a curve that seemed even larger now that it stood by itself. I looked strange and uneven and peculiar to myself, but somehow, ever so much more myself, and therefore so much more acceptable, than I looked with that thing

stuck inside my clothes. For not even the most skillful prosthesis in the world could undo that reality, or feel the way my breast had felt, and either I would love my body one-breasted now, or remain forever alien to myself.

Then I climbed back into bed and cried myself to sleep, even though it was 2:30 in the afternoon [p. 44].

Learning to value the breast that remains and mourning what is lost, while one is still in acute pain, are extremely difficult, as the following lines by Lorde (1980) show:

In playing back the tapes of those last days in the hospital, I found only the voice of a very weakened woman saying with the greatest difficulty and almost unrecognizable:

September 25th, the fourth day. Things come in and out of focus so quickly it's as if a flash goes by; the days are so beautiful now so golden brown and blue; I wanted to be out in it, I wanted to be glad I was alive, I wanted to be glad about all the things I've got to be glad about. But now it hurts. Now it hurts. Things chase themselves around inside my eyes and there are tears I cannot shed and words like cancer, pain, and dying [p. 45].

As she slowly recovers, Lorde attempts to integrate the two opposing forces that collide in the struggle with cancer. She tries to balance the death blow with a life force, and a new definition of her life, work, and body, slowly emerges: "The need to look death in the face and not shrink from it, yet not ever to embrace it too easily, was a developmental and healing task for me that was constantly being sidelined" (p. 47).

For Lorde, in her mid-40s and the mother of two daughters, and for Rollin, in her early 30s, the cancerous breast was never experienced as a sick, "bad" breast. Both women, who seemed to have had very good relationships with their bodies and with their mothers (internal object), emphasize that this "sick," lost breast was a good and beautiful one. Rollin (1978) writes:

I look at the empty place on my body and I get it, too. I get it.

A death in the body is, in some ways, like the other kind. One remembers the dead fondly. Sometimes the dead person seems more virtuous and wonderful than he or she was. I remember my left breast with love, real love. How I took it for granted! Isn't that silly; of course I took it for granted. Who goes around thinking, Gosh, lucky me to have two breasts.

Don't I take my other parts for granted?   Do I actively and devotedly appreciate my arms, my legs, my working brain? No. Not even now.

Difference between body-deaths and person-deaths: a person gets buried or burnt, ashes scattered, out of sight. The dead part of the body is destroyed too, of course, but the empty space remains. A widow can fill her dead husband's closets with her own clothing; she can fill the empty side of the bed with another man [p. 151].

Lorde (1980) tells us that her perception of her breast had already started to change during a four-week wait for the results of a biopsy (which turned out to be negative) a year before her illness was finally discovered:

> I had grown angry at my right breast because I felt as if it had in some unexpected way betrayed me, as if it had become already separate from me and had turned against me by creating this tumor which might be malignant. My beloved breast had suddenly departed from the rules we had agreed upon to function by all these years [p. 33].

But the day before her mastectomy, Lorde wrote in her journal,

> September 21, 1978
> The anger that I felt for my right breast last year has faded, and I'm glad because I have had this extra year. My breasts have always been so very precious to me since I accepted having them it would have been a shame not to have enjoyed the last year of one of them. And I think I am prepared to lose it now in a way I was not quite ready to last November, because now I really see it as a choice between my breast and my life, and in that view there cannot be any question [p. 34].

This affirmation of life, an identification with her good creative breast, wins the fight against her aggressive urges.

REPLACEMENT OF THE LOST BREAST WITH A NEW RELATIONSHIP

Another way of dealing with the loss of the breast is to replace the breast with a person, to start a new close relationship. This reaction has several facets. By changing partners, the mastectomized woman may be testing to see whether she is still sexually desirable. It may also be a way for her to assert her vitality. Starting a love affair can also be an act of aggression. The aggression seems primarily to emanate from the struggle against the malignant process, for one of the interesting features of these accounts is that the authors uniformly describe their husbands as supportive, loving, and helpful. Finally, starting the love affair at a time of great danger can be understood as acting out a *Liebestod* fantasy of Death as a lover, often illustrated in myth, fairy tales, and the arts. (Such fantasies are also frequently found in women with other terminal illnesses.) These four aspects usually coexist in every patient.

In Christine Lenker, a young married woman, we see most strongly the first aspect, the affirmation of femininity. Christine met a man at her first group therapy session. The man turned out to be a doctor from out of town who had come to the session because of a skin problem, not because of cancer. Soon after discussing their illnesses, they decided to leave the group and spend the time with each other. They developed a close, comfortable sensual and sexual relationship that lasted for several weeks until the doctor had to return home. Lenker (1984) writes, "I thought that the operations [mastectomy and ovariectomy] would take away my femininity, that I had to walk around as a neuter. . . (p. 52). A "neuter," for Lenker, was not only an asexual person, but also a thing that could not experience feelings of any kind. This affair helped Lenker to realize that she was still a woman, even with one breast, who could arouse and be aroused. Lenker described this short, fulfilling relationship as "the biggest miracle of my life, namely the sensation of a new femininity" (p. 50).

Rollin (1976) illustrates the aggressive aspect. After recovering from her mastectomy, Rollin felt increasingly uncomfortable in her marriage, even though she felt supported and sexually accepted. While she was in the hospital, an old friend, David, had made her a marriage proposal. One afternoon Rollin quickly packed and fled from New York to Philadelphia to her new lover: "What better time? There had been an earthquake in my life. . . . If I was going to do any major life renovation this was the time to do it, while everything was still a mess" (p. 198). She was amazed at the intensity of her husband's reaction—he loved her—and how he talked and wrote about the pain he experienced in losing her. The relationship with David ended abruptly when he pressed her to have a child by him, an act that would have entailed the danger of reactivating her cancer. Only after Rollin ran away from her lover too was she able to settle down emotionally to mourn her breast and to familiarize herself with her changed body and adopt a new outlook on life.

The enactment of a *Liebestod* fantasy can be seen in the following quotation. Shortly before her death, Hauri (1982) writes:

> The thought of approaching death is becoming seductive, it
> is exhilarating me; death gives me the possibility of a voyage
> and of an entire life change. . . . Tempting Death, you want to
> seduce me. Oh I know that you are standing on my doorstep:
> you are giving me reprieve [p. 27].

She imagines their union as reminiscent of the "oceanic feeling":

> And then, if I am lucky, I will be close to love in death, not
> to have to be alone. "Dying is beautiful," say those who believe
> they have already died once. I cling to their statements. How
> could I bear the future otherwise?   The fulfillment of all
> yearnings, weightless, bodiless, freedom, sunrise, morning—
> death is only a wakening, a morning [p. 69].

The idea of death as a lover appears in countless myths; for example,
in Greek mythology, Hades, the personification of death, is also depicted
as a dark and terrifying lover. In language, we speak of "the kiss of death"
and of "embracing death." In literature, perhaps the most famous example
is in Shakespeare. While Juliet lies drugged, Romeo says, "Ah, dear Juliet,
why art thou yet so fair?   Shall I believe that unsubstantial death is
amourous...." (V. iii, 101-103). In "The Theme of the Three Caskets," Freud
(1913b) analyzed the choice between three maidens, a typical motif in
myth and fairy tales, and developed the idea that the three represent the
three fates. Though of the three, the youngest is always the most desirable
one, she is also the goddess of death, with attributes, such as silence or
dumbness, that symbolically represent death, like Cordelia in *King Lear*. To
choose her is to choose death freely and not have it forced upon us, to
find death beautiful, not hideous, desired, not feared. These *Liebestod*
fantasies, libidinizing death as a partner, can be a source of comfort for the
dying woman (Greenberger, 1965).

This is how Reimann (1984), twice divorced, describes the first night
after mastectomy with her lover:

> The evening when he stayed over the first time, I told him
> that I was a woman cut in half. It was very difficult for me, but
> the shame and horror which I experience of myself disap-
> peared the moment he said that in the Orient, flaws were
> intentionally woven into especially beautiful carpets so that
> their perfection should not intimidate. A crazy comparison, but
> he thinks I am beautiful and complete, and he told me about
> those carpets fully relaxed, as if it were the most common

thing in the world to meet an amazon without being for a moment scared, dejected or pitying [p. 328].

Reimann succeeded with this new man, who seemed not to be frightened of a union in the face of death and stayed with him until her death.

THE PROJECTION OF AGGRESSION
IN WORKING THROUGH THE LOSS OF THE BREAST

One way of expressing aggression is to project it. Although projection may be uncomfortable for others, it is much better for the patient than introjection. Rollin (1976) describes it as follows:

> Anyway, people don't like "breast-cut-off" any more than they like "cancer." Breast-cut-off is too active, too descriptive. Breast-cut-off says what happens. And who wants to hear that, especially over a tuna fish sandwich? Why did I need to say it? I'm not sure. In a way, it was like vomiting. Perhaps I thought that if I kept spitting up I'd get rid of it and feel better. I did feel better. But then I'd feel worse almost right away again. So more throwing up. And more feeling better. And more feeling worse [p. 129].

Why did Rollin need to do it? To rid herself of some of the aggression that had accumulated while she was in the hospital playing the "Glad Girl," as she put it, acting tough and bravely accepting her surgeon's congratulations for having "such a good-looking wound" (see chapter 4). After her mastectomy, Hauri (1982) had proclaimed simply, "I hate people!" (p. 22). By contrast, Rollin (1978) saved her hatred for later, and even then she found an indirect way—"breast cut-off"—of discharging it.

> I told a lady at Kenneth who waxed my legs, a professor of mathematics at a cocktail party, and a saleswoman in the bathrobe department on the second floor of Bloomingdale's. I told Eugene. I told Beth Coolidge, a straight-talking and snooty-in-a-nice-way school chum from Boston whose response made my day: "My dear," she said in her most formidable lockjaw, "you will simply have to clutch one of those attractive little bags to your left side and keep it there." As solutions went, this was second only to Susan Wood's, who thought it would be nifty to get tattooed, "and then," she said, her mad, round little

eyes lighting up behind her mad, round little glasses, "I'll photograph you naked for Vogue" [p. 159].

When a cancer patient shoots out her aggression, she gets shot back!

BREAST CANCER AS SYMBOLIC IDENTIFICATION WITH THE BAD INNER IMAGE

Sometimes the tumor in the breast symbolizes a negative aspect of a significant person in the patient's life. This equivalence, however, is an unconscious one and surfaces only indirectly either in dreams or in artistic expression. There the patient's subjective fantasy can be expressed directly. The following example illustrates this process.

When she was only one and a half years old, Helen Webster, an American poet, lost her mother to breast cancer. A few years later, her older sister drowned. At 21, Webster herself developed breast cancer and was thus compelled to restructure her life. She became an artist and writer and took up scuba diving (perhaps unconsciously to search for her dead sister). Many years later, her cancer recurred. In the terminal stage of her illness, Webster wrote the following poem:

Child

Momma wants me
dead, drowned
like the kitten
in a bucket
held down
with sticks,
bloated
like my sister,
the smart one
the pretty one
the good one
who slipped
off a sailboat
in the sound,
floated in
twenty-one days
later.
Some days
I oblige her—

stop my ears
with mud
fill my mouth
with stones
plug my nose
with clay
block my eyes
with leaves
bind my body
with rags.
Then wait,
cocooned

—Webster (1980, p. 11)

In this poem, Webster describes her feeling that her mother was the transmitter of the deadly illness and with it death. Webster's breast cancer, as Meerwein (1988) has noted, is latently symbolized by this negative internal mother image. If in the poem one substitutes the word "cancer" for "Momma," one can see how the poet is describing her inner experience of the illness, which is in the process of killing her.

In the poem "To My Mother," by Claire Henze, we can feel the aggression against a callous, unempathic mother and an attempt to identify with a grandmother Henze never knew:

To My Mother

You told me the maid fainted
when she saw my grandmother
        in her bath.
Naked, upright, cheerful and witty
A terrible gash across her chest
No breasts.
And I picture the maid lying limp on
        the tile floor.
of this vast French bathroom,
my grandmother sitting in the big tub.
You say she was amused by the
        maid's shock,
and the picture doesn't hearten
or amuse or reveal her spirit,
or do anything but form a knot in my stomach
and make me weep.
My grandmother died long before I was born,
of the disease I have now.

I never knew her
but I know her now.
I know how she felt at that moment
when the maid fainted.
I know more about her now than
    anyone else.
And I know she was not amused.
           —Henze (1987, p. 48)

A similar split into a "good" grandmother-breast and a "bad" mother-breast can also be seen in the following poem by Murray:

Poem to My Grandmother in Her Death

After a dozen years of death
even love wanders off, old faithful
dog tired of lying on stiff marble.

In any case you would not understand
this life, the plain white walls
& the books, a passion lost on you.

I do not know what forced your life
through iron years into a shape of giving—
an apple, squares of chocolate, a hand.

There should have been nothing left
after the mean streets, foaming washtubs,
the wild cries of births at home.

Never mind. It's crumbling in my hands,
too, what you gave. I've jumped from ledges
& landed oddly twisted, bleeding internally.

Thus I learn how to remember your injuries—
your sudden heaviness as fine rain fell, or
your silence over the scraped bread board.

Finding myself in the end is finding you
& if you are lost in the folds of your silence
then I find only to lose with you those years

I stupidly flung off me like ragged clothes
when I was ashamed to be the child
of your child. I scrabble for them now

In dark closets because I am afraid.
I have forgotten so much. If I could meet you

again perhaps I could rejoin my own flesh

And not lose whatever you called love.
I could understand your silences & speak them
& you would be as present to me as your worn ring.

In the shadows I reach for the bucket of fierce
    dahlias
you bought without pricing, the coat you shook
free of its snow, the blouse that you ironed.

There's no love so pure it can thrive
without its incarnations. I would like to know you
once again over your chipped cups brimming with
    tea.
            —Murray (1975, p. 67)

The disowned negative mother image, which Murray inwardly identifies with, comes across clearly in the line "When I was ashamed to be the child of your child." Murray's cancer is closely connected—"to lose with you those years"—to that disavowed identification. At the same time, there is a strong wish to find the "good" grandmother as the poet moves closer to death.

    Picture 1, a drawing taken from a lengthy art psychotherapy treatment of a 39-year-old woman who suffered from breast cancer, illustrates

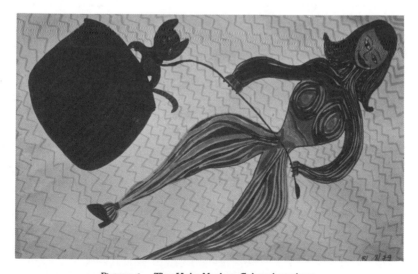

Picture 1. *The Holy Mother.* Colored markers.

the same strong split. According to the patient, she had intended to paint the "Holy Mother," and she was surprised to recognize in the images her own strong, phallic mother (with two breasts) and herself as the scared baby dog (without breasts) kept on a leash. At the time the patient drew this picture, her mother was taking care of her because she was paralyzed from the waist down because of a metastasis in her vertebrae. The picture also illustrates the two sides of the patient: her identifications, on one hand, with the strong, phallic mother, and, on the other, with the helpless, frightened nonbreasted, dependent self. This drawing allowed the patient to recognize the split she had felt after her mastectomy, which had left her with only one healthy breast, and to see how she divided her caretakers into good (breast) and bad (breast) by projection.

A more complex illustration of this split is to be found in Mrs. W, a 40-year-old mother of two children who was mastectomized because of breast cancer and who developed leukemia several years later. In the course of psychotherapy, during which she developed a close transference relationship with her therapist, she remembered for the first time her warm, loving grandmother, who had always given her special attention and singled her out for little gifts. This positive grandmother image stood in opposition to a "bad" image of the mother who could not care for or love her children but who nonetheless remained infuriatingly healthy with two intact breasts and a boyfriend. This internal split, not easily symbolized by a healthy "good" breast and a cancerous "bad" breast, was projected onto the nursing team and onto the therapist. The patient feared that her great envy of her healthy mother would destroy the relationship with the therapist and thereby threaten the truly "good" yet vulnerable breast of the internal grandmother image. Interpretation of this envy and the creation of a supportive relationship with the therapist made it possible for the patient to counterbalance the sick, and therefore "bad," breast with the introjection of the "good" healthy breast of the therapist-cum-grandmother (for a discussion of her envy, see chapter 13).

As we saw in the previous chapter, the good and bad objects can be more easily synthesized when there is "good enough mothering" (Winnicott, 1965) during the depressive position in infancy (Klein, 1948). As a result, the ego becomes more integrated, and hope for the reestablishment of a good object can be sustained in the face of ambivalence and loss. Because cancer and its threat of death also foster unconscious depressive anxieties, a repetition and continuation of the working-through process of the infantile depressive position is required. In infancy the child conquered internal chaos to establish a "good" internal object. So, too, with an acute life threat: a satisfactory adjustment to life with death depends on the same process.

When the balance of good and bad tends toward hatred of the

internal object, psychologically destructive forces, such as excessive narcissism, greed, envy, and grandiosity, rise to the foreground. Love and hate are split apart and bestowed on separate object images, as we saw in the poems by Webster and Murray and in the two case vignettes.

When the balance between love and hate tends toward love, then the unconscious memory of the residual hatred left over from the depressive position in infancy can be mitigated by love. Death and destruction can be tempered by creative reparation and a wish to live. If unconsciously the healthy breast has been physically and symbolically damaged by hate, it can be revived and healed again by loving grief. If envy of those who are healthy can be mitigated by an appreciation of what one has left and by confidence and hope for the future, rather than through continual denial, then pain, guilt, and grief for a lost perfection can be endured and overcome by an active attempt at reparation and symbolic "self-repair." Hauri (1982) expresses this need for active repair in terms both of her boundaries and of her sense of the future: "I have to create contours, I have no contours. . . . Illness means also to have a chance. I am provoked to think, to reflect, to change so the foe cancer has no opportunity to kill me" (p. 15). Lorde (1980) says much the same in a more clearly defined way, though she emphasizes the inner struggle involved:

> It was very important for me, after my mastectomy, to develop and encourage my own internal sense of power. I needed to rally my energies in such a way as to imagine myself as a fighter resisting rather than as a passive victim suffering. At all times, it felt crucial to me that I make a conscious commitment to survival. It is physically important for me to be loving my life rather than to be mourning my breast. I believe it is this love of my life and my self, and the careful tending of that love which was done by women who love. . . .
>
> In a perspective of urgency, I want to say now that I'd give anything to have done it differently—it being the birth of a unique and survival-worthy, or survival-effective, perspective. Or I'd give anything not to have cancer and my beautiful breast gone, fled with my love of it. But then immediately after I guess I have to qualify that—there really are some things I wouldn't give. I wouldn't give my life, first of all, or else I wouldn't have chosen to have the operation in the first place, and I did. I wouldn't give Frances, or the children, or even any one of the women I love. I wouldn't give up my poetry, and I guess when I come right down to it I wouldn't give my eyes, nor my arms. So I guess I do have to be careful that my urgencies reflect my priorities.

Sometimes I feel like I'm the spoils in a battle between good and evil, right now, or that I'm both sides doing the fighting, and I'm not even sure of the outcome nor the terms. But sometimes it comes into my head, like right now, what would you really give?   And it feels like, even just musing, I could make a terrible and tragic error judgement if I don't always keep my head and my priorities clear. It's as if the devil is really trying to buy my soul, and pretending that it doesn't matter if I say yes because everybody knows he's not for real anyway. But I don't know that. And I don't think this is all a dream at all, and no, I would not give up love [pp. 73-77].

Lorde's inner balance inclines strongly toward love, and her strength derives from her capacity to maintain that balance in the face of irrevocable loss: "The pain of separating from my breast was as sharp as the pain of separation from my mother. But I made it once before, so I know I can make it again" (p. 26). Lorde's good internal object is illustrated by the recollection that came to mind the day before her mastectomy and returned again in a dream the night after. Both the memory and the dream equipped her to deal with her loss and guided her toward creative reparation:

Eudora Garett . . . was the first woman who totally engaged me in our loving. I remember the hesitation and tenderness I felt as I touched the deeply scarred hollow under her right shoulder and across her chest the night she finally shared the last pain of her mastectomy with me. . . . Eudora came to me in my sleep . . . and we held hands for a while [p. 35].

The next day Lorde writes in her journal, "Eudora what did I give you? . . . Did you know how I loved you? You never talked of your dying, only of your work" (p. 36).

The creative product, whether book, poem, or picture, is unconsciously reintrojected and can thereby stimulate further creativity. Writing a book or a poem can thus be experienced as a life-giving enterprise that transforms the loss, with its fears of death, into an active, constructive experience. With the help of this creative product, the ultimate inevitability of death can be faced and accepted.

To the extent that women with breast cancer can, in their creations, once more work through the depressive position of infancy, they are able to regain a sense of wholeness and to become more confident of their capacity to love, more secure in their ability to mourn what has been lost, rather than hate or feel persecuted by it. Through projective and introjective identification with the "good creative breast," they learn to live with a limited but reliable feeling of emotional security, which is life.

━━ 11 ━━

Writing as Reparation
in the Face
One's Own Death

Literature written by cancer patients demonstrates how a heightened sense of omnipotence accompanied by a temporal suspension of reality enables author/patients to adapt to their life-threatening situation. By writing, cancer patients stay in touch with their fantasies and inner objects. They also balance past history with present reality and threatening future. If in this endeavor they also find a companion (doctor, therapist, or friend) with whom they can share their ongoing work, they can shield themselves from the terrible isolation and loneliness inherent in the fear of death. Creative writing and newly regained object constancy make cancer authors realize that they can still obtain narcissistic gratification despite the threat of death. New hope is fostered as they recover the sense of a life purpose that has been undermined by illness. Mourning their loss through writing, they are able to meet death with equanimity.

LOSS AND THE CANCER PATIENT

Psychologically speaking, cancer takes place deep within the "self" of the patient. The "self" is a partly conscious and partly unconscious inner representation of ourselves that we develop over the course of our lives. To a significant degree, it is made up of good as well as bad experiences that occur in early childhood in relation to our bodies, our person, and the significant others in our lives. Our sense of self-worth is largely determined by the quality of these early experiences and by our ability to work them through later in life. Psychological well-being is not possible without a sense of self-worth.

Both consciously and unconsciously, cancer often represents for the patient the bad part of his personality or his bad inner objects ("bad introjects"), and thereby directly influences his feelings about himself and his relationships with others.

Every cancer patient feels that his cancer intrudes from within. "I am being eaten up by my cancer," say many patients. Acting on an ancient dictum, deeply rooted in the earliest experiences of a body-self, the cancer patient responds by trying to empty his inner space so as to get rid of the bad introjects represented by his cancer. The result is that the patient tends to experience himself as empty precisely when he is most closely threatened by death. This can result in isolation and annihilation (Meerwein, 1987a). The danger is illustrated in the following account by Alsop (1973):

> Restlessly, I got up to do some exploring. I wandered about, and came to a door off the solarium, and pushed it open, and found myself in an auditorium.
>
> Then I saw the words that frightened me. There was a large placard on a stand, presumably for the indoctrination of newly arrived doctors and nurses. It was headed Rules for Admission, and there were ten or twelve numbered rules. I read only the first two: ALL PATIENTS MUST HAVE INCURABLE CANCER. ALL PATIENTS MUST BE INFORMED FRANKLY OF THEIR CASE.
>
> I turned around quickly and shut the door. I said nothing to Tish [his wife], except that I wanted to go back to the room. Somehow those printed words brought home the reality to me in a way that all John Glick's [the physician] kindly candor had not, and inside me there was a dark pit of fear [p. 51].

The confrontation with death forces the cancer patient to make tremendous inner changes. On a narcissistic level, there is first the mourning for the lost integrity of one's body, which continually and painfully disintegrates. If we remember that the earliest development of the ego is closely connected with the image of an intact body-ego, we can appreciate the threat to the feelings of self-worth that the patient experiences when his body disintegrates, as well as the strong feelings of shame and anger that follow in its wake. A poem by Helen Webster, who started to write after she first contracted breast cancer from which she later died, illustrates this point:

THE MIRROR

Startles
a stranger's face:
Bald imposter,
stunned, staring.
I ask:
Who are you?
Not I.
That young/old
plastic mask—
not mine.
The eyes,
perhaps,
I own.
They seem
surprised
by the stripped
skull,
The naked face
I deny.

      —Webster (1980, p. 38)

  The patient who is forced to withdraw libidinal cathexis from his body and thus from most of his drive wishes can do this satisfactorily only if he is able to cathect his inner experiences and fantasies more strongly than before. If he cannot make this transition, he often becomes inexorably depressed. The following poem illustrates the process well:

   Note from the Hospital

   Indulge me, please,
   I'm dying.
   Were you to
   see me bedded thus—
   leaking, drying,
   bagged, bruised,
   oozing, drugged,
   drained, tubed,
   maimed,
   slashed, sliced,
   stitched, stapled,
   shaved, stinking,

stuck—
I fear
our spider's web
of love
would tear;
a few strands
might cling,
but are easily
brushed away.
                    —Webster (1980, p. 89)

Webster is describing what it is like to be unable to go beyond a dying body because one cannot cathect the weak "spider's web of love." With her body attacked and dying, and her object relations so weakened that they might tear, she cannot revive her inner world. Only the patient who is able to make this transition becomes capable of mourning her sick, ailing body and reconciling herself to impending death.

On an object relational level, the mourning entailed in dying is necessarily accompanied by a continuous withdrawal of cathexis from people and things in the outer world. As part of this process, in the terminal phase the patient develops a strong wish to resolve his negative feelings toward his past and toward the people closest to him so as to take leave of them more easily. The better and the more supportive the inner and internalized experiences stemming from his early mother-child relationship, the easier it is for the patient to resolve his feelings as he begins to mourn the loss of his outer world. The more ambivalent those internalized relationships are, by contrast, the more difficult it is for the patient to experience a true feeling of mourning.

The following poem describes an identification with a bad internal mother image, which makes the process of mourning difficult:

A Haunting

My mother's hand is fiddling with the spoon
but my face, grown monstrous,
stares back at me from the bowl's tipsy reflection
before it ripples in the clear soup—
shattered!
Ah Madam my hand trembles.
Food spatters on the cloth,
food and the old terrors staining.
My mother's hand is breaking off the flowers.
Petal by petal they die

in the fierce grip of her hands.
My house is littered with dying flowers.
The stink of them fouls the gracious walls.

I dance on the lawn under the sun.
My shadow springs with me
lightly. . .
mine, mine!
My mother's feet are crushing the grass
in my dance.
All of us pregnant with our ghosts.
                              —Murray (1974, p. 11)

In the lines, "My house is littered with dying flowers" and "All of us are pregnant with our ghosts," we find a symbolic identification of the malignant cancer with the negative mother image.

Much of the cancer literature discussed in this chapter focuses on the reparation of the cancer sufferer's multitudinous losses.

THE TEMPORAL SUSPENSION OF REALITY
FOR THE SAKE OF ADAPTATION AND CREATION

In "Fear of Breakdown," written shortly before his death, Winnicott (1974) lists the "primitive agonies" of the patient who fears breaking down: "1. a return to an unintegrated state; 2. falling forever; 3. loss of psychosomatic collusion, failure of indwelling; 4. loss of sense of reality" (p. 104). All of the cancer-authors appear to experience the same overwhelming fears that Winnicott describes. So where do they find the strength and creative energy to write their books? In part, the ability of the cancer patients to write reflects a simple denial of their danger, but that is not the whole story.

While he was mourning his beloved wife and at the same time dying of cancer himself, the American psychoanalyst Ping Ni Pao wrote "The Suspension of the Reality Principle in Adaptation and Creativity," which was published posthumously in 1983. It describes how a person in a threatening situation can extend his sense of omnipotence and so suspend reality for a short time without cutting himself off from reality entirely. Our cancer-authors also seem to have developed just such a heightened sense of their own magical power to suspend reality, enabling them to believe that they could control the threat through their writing. This new sense of omnipotence was a psychic prerequisite, frequently unconscious, for undertaking and completing their creative endeavors.

The following two rather grandiose quotations illustrate the sense of omnipotence that may suddenly emerge in the face of death. The first is from Peter Noll (1987): "Soon after the diagnosis I had the redeeming thought that my death should be celebrated, maybe already the span between the onset of the tumor and death, surely however after my death" (p. 12). The second quotation is by Walter Matthias Diggelmann (1979), who suffered from a brain tumor:

> If my slow dying, which can no longer be denied, is predestined, then I have only one last wish. That I might make out of this dying a grand, beautiful interesting story, a story which would make so much money that I could study medicine, neurology, and build a hospital so I could invent a brain. I would invent a brain for an inventor who invents inventors and who tells those inventors he invented what they would have to invent in the future. I would thus be the inventor of the inventor's inventor. I would be the inventor of myself [p. 28].

The loss of the feeling of self-worth and the impairment and partial loss of the body-ego provoke enormous fear and suffering. In the face of this acute threat, the patient longs for his previous intact state. Unconsciously, he longs for his earliest sense of completeness when he was united with his protective first object. In creative writing, the author can relinquish part of his conscious defenses and slide into a creative regression in the service of his ego; in the depths of this regression he can breathe new life into his lost, destroyed, and beloved object. In the written product, moreover, the cancer patient can find a new gestalt, which fosters new, satisfying feelings that give conscious testimony to the inner revival of and union with the primary object. To put it differently, through the power of his fantasies in conjunction with his activity, the patient can stabilize his badly damaged dynamic and libidinal-economic balance.

This new balance perhaps can be best illustrated by a remarkable passage from Fitz Mullan (1985), in which he describes his successful fight against his lung tumor. His unabashed fantasy of fusion—of returning to the womb—helped Mullan survive the immediate life threat:

> At one point when I was at my sickest and most desperate, I developed a vivid and urgent fantasy about returning to the womb. The problem lay there, I told myself, and the only true solution rested in returning to the site of the crime and starting all over again. Chemotherapy and radiation were after the fact

and relatively useless. I felt like Humpty Dumpty with all the king's horses and all the king's men trying to mend me.

As I lay in bed struggling against nausea, my eyes wandering aimlessly over the input and output charts taped to the walls. . . . I imagined starting all over again. It seemed so logical and so hopeful. This has all been a terrible mistake and it's ending so absurdly that we must simply stop and begin again. How, I wondered, would I get back inside? I was so damned big—so embarrassingly huge. And would Mom really want to go through it all again? She would have to participate. I knew I couldn't do it alone. Would she be willing to put up with another labor and delivery and a toddler and school and measles and all that over again? I felt she could be persuaded if she understood why, but the size problem was a real one. How would I ever get back inside? For days, through my worst bouts of nausea and depression, unable to eat and scared beyond reason, with Mom present and not present, I was obsessed with my return to the womb. This fantasy, wild as it was, helped me through some awful times. When all my rationality as a physician, as a patient, as a son told me that I was cornered, it gave me a way out. Gradually, as the worst effects of the therapy wore off and as the possibility of life reemerged, the fantasy became less frequent and less compelling [pp. 45-46].

In a similar vein, Beutler (1980) describes how she was able to retrieve her inner fantasies and inner objects and thereby control her fear. Her fantasies also illustrate her wish to fuse with the once omnipotent father who had suffered from the same neck carcinoma that she had, but who lived actively to old age. By creatively working through her fears and losses, Beutler is acting on her father's advice: "Don't just cry if the world doesn't suit you. Put it over your knees and spank it till it moves around again" (p. 67). The following quotation describes Beutler's fear and fantasy when she awakens after her neck operation and in terror finds that she is unable to talk or move her tongue:

Father, father—why do you call? Rocks are in my mouth and I cannot move them. . . . Here I am father—I'm pushing myself against these rocks. I am incarcerated in bones . . . , I am masoned into the earth? . . . Father is in the house. Do you promise? [Mother] I don't have to struggle any more, you see. The door flies open; my mother waits seeing, and my father is in the house . . . [p. 78].

Ted Rosenthal tries to surmount his fear of death by hoping to find "the real lost love;" he was only 31 years old, suffering from acute leukemia, when he wrote the following lines:

> I cannot turn it off
> Cannot be naked
> Cannot go away
> I pace madly, flop in bed, sit hunched
> Vaguely applauding
> Thinking time for inspiration, and dreaming
> Of love—
> What place for me
> In this pioneer steel-jawed daring rush North
> To plow heart and free treasures
> From ice clenched fist of self?
> I must pull myself together.
> I must go!
> To leap past prayers come I North
> Unprepared breathing madly,
> Wondering about my soul and the real lost love
> To find.
>   —Rosenthal (1973, p. 21)

In an empty world of grief, fear, and terror, the writing patient can cathect a fantasy that fills up his inner emptiness and enriches his external existence. The three preceding statements demonstrate impressively how important it is for the cancer patient to keep in touch with his fantasies. Death is the ultimate being alone, the irreversible separation from mother, but psychologically it includes the mitigating fantasy of a union with her as Mother Earth (Freud, 1913b, p. 301).

Dora Hauri (1982) illustrates her wish for fusion with the earth when she writes,

> Barefoot I walked over the freshly ploughed field. With bare feet I touched the earth. I was the fall, flowers and leaves being used from the summer, sun wind and rain, they fall, change colors, they want to be looked at in their yellow and red, falling, I saw fall. I walked with bare feet over the field [p. 33].

Fantasies and dreams help the patient to maintain the integrity of his self and thus avert unbearable loneliness and terror. Diggelmann (1979) puts it like this:

Why not invent a story: "The Man with the Wicked Tree in His Head"? Something will come to mind; I will die only if I can no longer invent something. I am dead when I no longer invent anything. I am dead when I am silent [p. 62].

Writing is also the means by which cancer patients maintain an active dialogue with their past, present, and future. It enables them to regain a sense of the balance of the "seasons" of life that have been shaken and clouded through their fears. Sikes (1988), who suffers from breast cancer, describes how her sense of time has changed since she was confronted with a life threatening disease:

When I was young, time seemed endless. To wait to run flying from school at the end of the day, to wait until he deigned to look at me, to wait was impossible. Time wouldn't pass.

Now Time is impossible too, but it's different. I no longer wait for it. I have to run to catch up. I try to seize it, force it to slow down hold it still for a moment, but I cannot. Now I am like the child traveling in a car who tires of looking forward and begins to stare out the back window at the road unrolling behind her. "Slow down," she shouts, "I *saw* something!"

But she is not in control and the car has hurtled ahead. The vision is lost.

We are always children [pp. 80-81].

Cancer patients often feel that they have lost their sense of time. As Diggelmann (1979) writes in his hospital diary, "It is the strange feeling that my sense of time has changed. Time passes very slowly, like sand through an hourglass" (p. 63). The sense that cancer patients have of being trapped in the ebb of time is described by Ted Rosenthal as he lies in the hospital with acute leukemia:

What has this reckless stab of life to do with me
and my mud thoughts?
Over thirty in search of vitality
Lonely, longing, yearning
Afraid to give anything up
Tired Earthbound I, am I to leap North
Ultimate North
Siberia fur trade North where all sound
Turns to roaring crackling noise

In the transcontinental trap
Of time?

—Rosenthal (1973, p. 20)

The sense of disintegration—"mud thoughts" in a world of "roaring, crackling noise"—that comes through in this poem is related to the cancer patient's loss of touch with time's natural rhythms.

Cancer patients who lose their sense of time also lose their sense of life security. Thus, in writing and creation, they do everything in their power to maintain a sense of time. Noll (1984), for instance, made special efforts to follow the movement of time. He suffered from carcinoma of the bladder, which he refused to treat medically. In his journal the changing seasons are described as he observed them on a little mountain lake outside his cottage where he retreated to write. His observation and recording of the seasonal changes gave Noll a hold on the little time he had left to live. The image of the lake and its transformations recurs throughout his diary, like a recurrent melody in a larger work. The movement of the seasons provided Noll with a comforting connection to the continuity of the waters of life. It also served as a mirror reflecting the projected image of his own passing:

December 28th, 1981
... My look is directed towards the oversnowed lake and the forest behind, from the pine trees snow is falling. . . [p. 7].

January 22nd, 1982
The dark forest behind the snowy little lake and the white slope towards Falera are very beautiful, I would like to see them all a long time yet [p. 14].

May 27th, 1982
The little lake has grown big; its water is now muddy, brown green. From every direction, birds are singing to me. . . . The cuckoo is calling from afar proclaiming the idea of an early summer. Spring I missed, if it took place [p. 198].

July 9th, 1982
Two herons descend on the edge of the little lake; for the first time I hear their strong, ugly screams [p. 237].

July 10th, 1082
... when I look outside I feel a totally new experience, as though the Earth is rolling away from the sun and towards the

stars. In the morning this feeling is not with me. It is an evening sensation [p. 238].

July 24th 1982
   The little lake is now beautifully overgrown by reeds. The lake is also nice in the rain which covers the forest with a fine veil [p. 243].

August 27th 1982
   It turned cold. It is raining with a dozing, silent noise into the foggy twilight. The little lake is now all overgrown. But the reed is still green [p. 258].

Noll saw nature according to his inner perception. In his weakened state, he felt death approaching. His earth really did roll slowly away toward heaven, toward the evening and toward the dark. It was he who was living in a "foggy twilight."

"CREATIVITY TRANSFERENCE" OR THE "GIFT SITUATION" BETWEEN CANCER/AUTHOR AND COMPANION

Before the cancer/author actually begins to write, he fantasizes about writing. It is then, at this preliminary stage, that his feelings of omnipotence seem to be especially powerful. The sense of omnipotence propels him to create and allows him the illusion that through his writing he can prevent impending disaster. When he starts to write, his focus shifts from his omnipotence to his inner self, leading to isolation. Added to this is the isolation that everyone who is threatened by death experiences.

In loneliness and isolation, the cancer/author has an especially strong need to feel close to a supportive companion, someone close with whom he can share his creation. With this companion, the cancer/author has a kind of idealized transference relationship, similar to the one between any dying patient and his psychiatrist or psychotherapist. In this relationship, both partners experience an intense giving and receiving, which is stimulated by a regressive wish for an early idyll of love, security, and total trust.

This kind of close relationship has also been described by many healthy artists (Auchter, 1978). Kohut (1975) calls it a "creativity-transference" and describes it as an idealized transference that derives from a normal phase of development in which the child's experiences of the empathic adult as omnipotent evokes in the child a feeling of confidence and narcissistic well-being. Kohut describes how during creative activity artists often find for themselves a person whom they consider omnipotent and with whom they can temporarily fuse. Earlier, Eissler (1955/1973) described a similarly close, idealized relationship between the dying patient and his psychiatrist; Eissler termed this a "gift-situation." The "gift" for the patient can be his therapist, doctor, or companion as the available object.

The cancer/author typically chooses a person, not infrequently his physician, who can satisfy the omnipotent transference and who is available so that the author can temporarily fuse with him or her. Or else the person selected may be a friend, family member, or role model. Maxi Wander (1980) described the essential process succinctly in her September 25, 1976 journal entry: "I wrote to Christa W. [Wolf, a very famous East German writer] in Vienna. I would like her to come, so that I can nurse myself on her life. Life transfusion" (p. 31).

Another illustration of this point is the case of Ulysses S. Grant, 18th President of the United States. Seven years after leaving office, in 1884, Grant was a ruined man, his career destroyed and his business bankrupt. He had also fallen ill of a squamous-cell carcinoma of the neck, the poor prognosis of which his exceptional physician, Dr. Hancock Douglas, kept him very well informed. In this state, Grant was visited by Mark Twain, a great admirer. Twain suggested that Grant write his memoirs, which he would publish by his own publishing company, Webster and Co.; Twain was willing to pay a large sum of money in advance. Grant, who was in incredible pain from his no longer operable carcinoma and who had never written more than a few letters, accepted this rather unrealistic proposal. Grant's principal motive was to provide financial security for his family after his death. Mark Twain was just then being celebrated for his novel, *Huckleberry Finn*, and the author's confidence in Grant's literary abilities, combined with the outstanding support of Grant's devoted doctor, made it possible for Grant to write his two-volume autobiography, despite his pain and weakness. With the help of his two companions, Grant was able to recathect the self-confidence that had been so badly injured by his terrible illness and financial failures. The renewal of his sense of omnipotence enabled him to suspend temporarily the reality of his dying. He died five days after finishing the second volume of his autobiography, on the day he himself had predicted. He died surrounded by his family and physician. Grant's memoirs are comparable to the commentaries written by Julius Caesar, and expert consensus is that his writings have great historical and literary value (Nelson, 1981).

The full trust extended him by Twain and his doctor, Hancock

Douglas, provided Grant with what Winnicott (1971) termed a "holding environment." The resultant feeling of being held and supported fostered new hope and made it possible for him to rebalance past, present, and future. The last letter Grant addressed to his physician (in Nelson, 1981) shows that once he had finished his two volumes, nothing remained that could provide a hold on to life:

> Dr., since coming to this beautiful climate and getting a complete rest for about ten hours, I have watched my pains, and compared them with those of the past few weeks. I can feel plainly that my system is preparing for dissolution in one of three ways: one by hemorrhage; one by strangulation; and the third by exhaustion. The first and second are liable to come at any moment to relieve me of my earthly sufferings. The time of arrival of the third can be computed with almost mathematical certainty. With an increase in daily food, I have fallen off in weight and strength very rapidly in the past two weeks. There cannot be hope of going far beyond this period [p. 435].

Another example of a creativity transference is the relationship between Alice James and her friend and companion Katharine Peabody Loring, as described in the diary James kept during the last three years of her life. Even though the friendship between the two women had begun about 11 years earlier, it became much more important for the sickly James during those final years. When, in the last year of her life, Alice James was diagnosed with terminal breast cancer, the strong bonds with Katharine helped her to overcome her anxiety and pain and enabled her to continue to write, until the day before she died.

Four months before her death, James (1964) wrote in her diary:

> Three or four weeks ago the treacherous friend Morphia which while murdering pain, destroys sleep and opens the door to all hideous nervous distresses, disclosed its iniquities to us, and K [Katharine Peabody Loring] and I touched bottom more nearly than ever before [p. 222].

One month later, another note in her diary reads:

> As the ugliest things go to the making of the fairest, it is not wonderful that this unholy granite substance in my breast should be the soil propitious for the perfect flowering of Katharine's unexampled genius for friendship and devotion.

The story of her watchfulness, patience and untiring resource cannot be told by my feeble pen, but all the pain and discomfort seem a slender price to pay for all the happiness and peace with which she fills my days [p. 225].

The day before she died, James dictated to Miss Loring her last entry:

May 4th 1892
  I am being ground slowly on the grim grindstone of physical pain, and on two nights I had almost asked for K's lethal dose, but one steps hesitantly along such unaccustomed ways and endures from second to second, and I feel sure that it can't be possible but what the bewildered little hammer that keeps me going will very shortly see the decency of ending his distracted career; however this may be, physical pain however great ends in itself and falls away like dry husks from the mind, whilst moral discords and nervous horrors sear the soul. These last, Katharine has completely under the control of her rhythmic hand, so I go no longer in dread of the wonderful moment when I feel myself floated for the first time into the deep sea of divine cessation, and saw all the dear old mysteries and miracles vanish into vapour! . . .
  Katharine can't help it, she's made that way, a simple embodiment of Health, as Baldwin [James Mark] called her "The New England Professor of doing things [p. 232].

Katharine Loring's commentary shows us how important this entry was for the dying James. James could not relax before she had expressed her gratitude for Katharine's devotion to her, this while honoring her as a "Professor," in keeping with her sardonic style, which runs all through her diary. Katharine Loring (in James, 1964) writes, "The dictation of March 4th was rushing about in her brain all day, and although she was very weak and it tired her much to dictate, she could not get her head quiet until she had it written: then she was relieved . . ." (p. 232). Only after thanking her beloved friend for the beautiful "gift" she had received could James die in peace.

An equally strong "creativity transference" can be found in Peter Noll's (1984) *Dictations on Death and Dying.* Three days after the diagnosis of his bladder carcinoma and his decision not to treat it, Noll met with his good friend, the famous Swiss author Max Frisch, and asked him to give the funeral oration after his death in the Grossmuenster Church in Zurich. Frisch agreed and thus began his role as the companion who supported Noll on his last way. The strong identification and close friendship with the famous author gave Noll the strength and inspiration to write his impressive book in the face of the constant threat of death. Early in the illness, they even traveled together to Egypt. Later on, the sicker Noll became, the more important were his friend's visits and their intellectual conversations. At one point, when Noll spent a few days alone at a resort, he began doubting the quality of his dictations and became depressed. Then, sadly, during the terminal stage of the illness, Frisch had to travel abroad. The friends said goodbye, and before Frisch landed at his destination, Noll had died.

FRITZ ZORN: WRITING AS A PHALLIC DEFENSE

I would like to end with a negative example of the thesis advanced in this chapter—the psychological self-portrait found in the book *Mars* by the Swiss cancer/author Fritz Zorn, a graduate of Zurich University with a degree in Romance languages. Written in 1977, *Mars* became a best-seller and a symbol, indeed a manifesto, for an entire generation; it has been translated into many languages. I will not discuss here the book's psychosocial or sociopolitical messages nor the author's thesis that cancer is psychological in origin. Rather, I will focus on the parts that are relevant to the issues of creativity and reparation.

Zorn opens his work with the following declaration:

> I am young, rich and well educated, and I am unhappy, neurotic and alone. I come from one of the best families on the right side of the Lake of Zurich, called the "Gold Coast". We are middle class and I have been nice all my life. . . . Naturally I also have cancer, the logical result of the above mentioned words . . . [p. 23].

This statement is not an act of overcoming grief, but a reiteration of the author's sense of hopelessness. Zorn describes how he grew up and experienced childhood without having been a child, adolescence without having been an adolescent, and adulthood without having attained maturity. The rigid rituals in his parent's home forced on him a total suppression of emotion. "The version of Hamlet's question that threatened my parents' home was: 'To live in harmony or not to live,'" he tells us (p. 28). The logical result of this emotional vacuum was Zorn's cancer, which finally relieved him of years of depression, first latent, later manifest. In his cancer he found a foe he could fight, and in fighting, he found an identity. The name Zorn, meaning anger in German, is a pseudonym; his real name was Angst, which means fear. In his book he finally gave vent to his anger; he began to strike out with the same deadly force that had struck him. Finally, he demanded to be heard.

Throughout adolescence Zorn had gone about with the feeling that "a dead crow was hanging from my neck" (p. 89), an uncanny premonition of his malignant lymphoma, which first manifested itself as a tumor of the neck. Zorn ruefully interpreted the tumor as all the swallowed tears that he could not cry and that had collected in his throat to form his deadly growth. *Mars* is a protest against this emotional death in life, the lamentation of a "puer" who at 31 had never experienced either emotional closeness or sexual love.

But, *Mars* is an autistic book. The author gives few details about his personal relationships. In more than 200 pages he never mentions that he had a brother, for example, nor does he mention the high school students he taught. He expresses no feelings other than disappointment, depression, hopelessness—and anger. Lamenting neither his lost objects, nor his past, nor his ailing body, nor the future that was cut short by his illness, he makes no attempt to mourn. The only emotively conveyed experience in the entire book comes at the end, and it is a vision of violence, a fantasy against his mother: "I kept seeing myself again and again pushing my mother down the cellar steps and watching her bloody head hit the stone floor again and again till the formless mass was reduced to a pool of blood. A gruesome vision—but a potent one" (p. 194).

This fantasy is followed by a second vision of exploding the Swiss bank where he had put the money he inherited from his father: "In this place lies my parental inheritance in a visual form. Least important, it contains thousands of francs; but more important it contains thousands of fears, miseries and despairs" (p. 195).

With these two visions, Zorn destroys his primary objects in fantasy. If there is little belief that the good object can be restored, either on the outside or on the inside, if it is felt as irretrievably lost, destroyed, persecuted, and persecutory—then the internal situation is inevitably felt as hopeless (Segal, 1964). Accordingly, the only protections from total despair that remain available to the author are violent defense mechanisms. Yet, the visions also illustrate Zorn's continuing identification with the lost and destroyed objects, for he hits as he has been hit. The feelings of triumph, contempt, and omnipotence that permeate this book are expressions of these violent defense mechanisms. Unlike the confidence born of a reunion with the good object, they do not serve to suspend temporarily the threatening reality that pervades Zorn's account. Zorn needs his book, and the rage that suffuses it, to build a wall around himself so as to distance his other emotions, to defend himself from feeling loss and grief, and to protect himself from feeling how insatiable are his overwhelming longings for closeness.

On an unconscious level, writing this book signifies for Zorn the reparation and reconstruction of his narcissistic integrity rather than the reparation of the lost inner object. In this sense, *Mars* illustrates the dynamic of phallic creativity described by Hagglund (1978, p. 125) and discussed earlier. The sense of vitality that accrues from the endeavor depends ultimately on a denial of loss at the deepest level, the implicit, unconscious assumption being that whatever goodness the lost object might have possessed is better regained through self-repair and the associated triumph over castration anxiety. Paradoxically, in a manner similar to that described by Chasseguet-Smirgal (1984b) in her study of perversion, this self-aggrandizement requires that Zorn also redirect his sadistic drives toward himself. In his book, Zorn unilaterally turns himself into a "case," thereby distancing himself farther from his human condition. Moreover, toward the end of the book he apotheosizes this situation by depicting himself as a fallen angel fighting God, a contest whose outcome can only be damnation. Zorn's creation ultimately does not help him to regain a feeling of self, but he does manage to experience a feeling of importance. As Muschg (1981) puts it in his comments on Zorn's book, "A feeling of omnipotence floats over his powerlessness or impotence; the grandiose mask covers up the fact that he has no face" (p. 72).

We read in Zorn's book that he went back into psychotherapy, which he had first attempted in adolescence. In so doing, he made an active attempt to find a partner to share his last journey, but to no avail. Zorn writes about his year of psychotherapy:

> It was the worst year of my life then; before I could create something new, everything had to be destroyed. . . . During that year I suffered incredible psychic torments, a factual dying, the death of my entire ego. In the end, this ego was totally dead and nothing was left of it [p. 143].

We read nowhere about the great feelings of disappointment and anger Zorn must have experienced over the futility of his attempt to share his life with somebody and to learn to communicate his needs at the last moment. Employing the same term with which his parents had cut off the uncomfortable questions he had asked as a child, Zorn writes that to describe psychotherapy would be "too difficult." It would have indeed been "too difficult" to admit that psychotherapy merely repeated his earliest trauma—the lack of emotional contact. And it likewise would have been too difficult to analyze the fatal, unconscious identification of both therapeutic partners with the destroyed inner object and, accordingly, with the cancer.

Mars described how his psychotherapy had only uncovered his incredible misery, his total lack of human contact, his great social isolation, and his impotence, resulting in his deep depression and sense of anomality. This projective identification by both therapeutic partners with the patient's "bad" introject symbolized in the cancer and consequent fusion with this "bad" introject, had augmented the patient's fear of extinction. His wish to empty himself of these bad introjects through psychotherapy left him with a total inner emptiness and at the same time with the dread of death. This identification is also impressively illustrated in the section where Zorn talks about his hatred of God and his powerful need for God to die: "I saw myself already involved in a fight with God, where we both used the same weapon, both used cancer. I am God's Carcinoma" (pp. 218-219).

This is not a union with a receiving Mother Earth nor with a protective Father God, but an identification with the bad part of the inner object and with his cancer. With this identification, death provides no relief. It is obvious that in this situation no "creativity transference" can develop, and there is no gift to be received. Fortunately, Zorn was able to make himself a gift in the form of this book, whose acceptance for publication he received via his psychotherapist the evening before his death. The following quotation illustrates the great need the book satisfied in Zorn:

> My suffering remains unchanged; the only thing I can do with this misery is to write it down again and again. As long as there is no relief to my pain I must keep proclaiming and crying out my misery, even though I cannot spew it out in its entirety. ... There is nothing beautiful about vomiting one's undigested past, but not to be able to vomit that past is even worse. The sickening feeling before the vomiting is still more uncomfortable than the vomiting itself [p. 184].

Considered apart from its dynamic functions, Zorn's creativity remains impressive. The author was able to turn the process of his physical and psychological destruction into a work of art. Projecting his narcissistic rage into the totality of his book, he regained a new, potent gestalt. Unfortunately it did not prevent him from being isolated, lonely, and very frightened of the prospect of his death:

> I have to die isolated and alone. . . . My fears and pains belong only to me, they cannot be abolished by my explaining them. . . . Many will understand why I am dying, but in that dying I am alone [p. 213]

SUMMARY

Just as cancer typically represents the "bad" parts of oneself—at the deepest level the degradations of the bad object—the threat of terminal cancer tends to be experienced psychologically in terms of the ultimate ascension of the bad object and the corresponding destruction of all goodness. Against this psychological threat, creativity, embodied in a final book, is a potent weapon. Through the heightened sense of omnipotence and the temporal suspension of reality inherent in the creative process, the author threatened by cancer can make reparation to his good objects and immortalize them in the form of his book. Since these objects are also part of his inner world, the author can regain a sense of a benign embeddedness in his past and reconstruct and repair his lost or destroyed loved objects. He can stay connected to them while writing and so mourn the world he is losing. During the process of writing, further, a close emotional relationship with a companion with whom he can temporarily fuse, and with whom he can share his creation, can enable the cancer patient to reclaim the present despite his bleak future and so rediscover a purpose in life to sustain him through his last days.

12

CLINICAL CONSIDERATIONS IN ART PSYCHOTHERAPY WITH CANCER PATIENTS

One might think that art therapy with cancer patients, some of whom are terminally ill, would be quite depressing, but this is not the case. The therapist is granted the same kind of creative protection as the reader of a cancer story. In addition, the therapist's own creative talent can sometimes help in working through particularly difficult countertransferential constellations.

As we saw in Chapter 9, Winnicott (1971) observed that between the fourth and sixth months of life children are able to create objects that they can regard as substitutes for mother. Winnicott considered this an act of primary creativity. He called the invested object a transitional object because it functions in the baby's transition from a primary union with the mother to a more independent self separate from other. With the help of the transitional object, the child is able to express separation anxieties in play and so overcome them.

We can observe an analogous process in art psychotherapy. There, we stage a meeting between the subjective world of the patient and external reality represented by the art therapist. The picture exists in the area between the two realms, a transitional space, and becomes a transitional object, a bridge between the inner and the outer world. Both worlds contribute to the creation of the picture. It is the picture that helps the patient to keep inner and outer reality simultaneously separated yet interrelated. As Otto Rank (1932/1968) wrote, "Art and play link the world of subjective unreality and objective reality, harmoniously fusing edges but not confusing them" (p. 104).

Through their pictures, patients express tangible and comprehensible projections of their inner images. The created picture can then be investigated and interpreted with the therapist. This particular kind of "experiencing together" provides psychological support within the protected confines of the creative process and facilitates a mutuality between patient and therapist. A primary partnership develops similar to the relationship between the playing child and its available, yet unobtrusive, mother. The patient can express his separation anxieties by painting, and the therapist can demonstrate his relatedness to the patient by accepting these anxieties and mirroring them back, thereby enabling the patient to reintroject them, that is, to assimilate them as part of a genuinely supportive experience. More deeply, the patient can overcome his separation anxieties by introjecting the therapist as a good object who is bonded to him. For both patient and therapist, the drawings created in the course of this process represent the bond between them.

The bond has another aspect. Beyond the patient's introjections of the therapist, the patient's creation of a painting that will survive his death makes it possible for the therapist to keep the bond alive even after the patient's demise; the painting will forever after remind the therapist of the patient. Hence, the picture becomes representative of the patient's fantasies of immortality. The fear of death, which all cancer patients experience independent of the prognosis of their illness, can be lessened by the hope of surviving in their creations (which reflect the total personality) and so living on in the memory of others.

Through his creations, the person threatened by death can express his strong emotions, especially those like jealousy and anger which would otherwise be repressed or denied. Because the therapist is able to recognize and mirror these split-off feelings, he makes them accessible to be worked through and integrated. The patient can relinquish his defenses against these emotions because he experiences the therapist as a good, intact object that his negative feelings cannot destroy. The resulting sense of emotional freedom can facilitate the task of self-repair. All cancer patients experience their illness as a threat to their sense of self, as a narcissistic lesion. Art therapy attempts, as one of its principal tasks, to reveal the intact, healthy, creative parts of the self, disclose them to the patient, and thus heal the rift.

Art therapy, as we see in the case studies that follow, is, however, not independent of the vicissitudes of the therapeutic relationship. Within a surprisingly short period of time, transference emerges, creating new links between patient and therapist. The emergence of transference means that the therapist is now invested with the various wishes, anxieties, and hopes—with the feelings of love, envy, and jealousy—that previously were associated with persons who played significant roles in the crucial periods of the patient's development. What makes the psychotherapeutic relationship with the cancer patient distinctive, however, is that these transference manifestations, expectable in any psychotherapy, are decisively colored by the psychological ramifications of the disease process. In what follows we will be looking more closely at the interpersonal dynamics associated with two kinds of cancer patients, those suffering from solid tumors and those suffering from leukemia.

ART PSYCHOTHERAPY WITH PATIENTS SUFFERING FROM LEUKEMIA

Since the entire body is affected by the malignant process of the disease, the patient suffering from leukemia is unable to localize his illness in any particular part of his body. Patients who suffer from leukemia, therefore, are subject to very intense fears that tend to flood them in the acute phase. Many factors are responsible for the overwhelming intensity of the patients' fears. These include the high fever and the debilitating physical weakness that are part of the illness, symptoms that make denial and rationalization impossible and that presage impending mortality. These symptoms, the global quality of their fears, and the resulting dread of psychic disintegration all conspire to make leukemia patients feel like weak and broken personalities. Accordingly, they tend to have powerful but ambivalent wishes of effecting a psychic reunion with the lost, good object, and they seek to make a reattachment to it via the external world, namely, by establishing a protected, secure, significant relationship with someone else.

The leukemia patient thus tends to see in the psychotherapist the embodiment of the totality of the healthy parts of himself (Dreifuss and Meerwein, 1984a). Consequently, he unconsciously wishes to unite psychologically with the therapist. The wish, however, frightens him, since such a merger would threaten his psychic integrity and undermine his independence, both of which have already been significantly diminished by the regression forced on the patient by his illness. Therefore, the leukemia patient has a great need to deny these wishes and to maintain a suitable inner distance from the therapist. The picture, located between the patient and the art therapist and serving as a transitional object, can help guarantee this urgently required distance. The picture helps the leukemia patient to avoid fusion with the therapist and thus to preserve a measure of autonomy. In addition, a sequence of pictures can serve as a means of monitoring possible disturbances in the relationship with the therapist and thus facilitates the maintenance of a working alliance between the two.

The following cases illustrate the various significances of art therapy for the person suffering from leukemia.

CASE 1

Mrs. S is a 58-year-old woman, the mother of two adult sons, hospitalized with AML (acute myelocytic leukemia). She had worked as a charwoman in a school until shortly before her illness began. I started to work with her when her hospital roommate, another patient of mine who was also suffering from leukemia, realized how much Mrs. S wanted contact with me and introduced us.

In the first picture (Picture 1), created spontaneously by the patient in the first session, we see several pairs of flowers. One flower in each pair, however, is in some way inferior: smaller, incomplete, or missing a petal. The pairs are thus composed of a healthy, strong member and a weaker, sick, incomplete one. We can hypothesize that the patient will exhibit an unconscious need to project her healthy self, free of illness, onto the healthy therapist, since she can no longer recognize it in herself (Dreifuss, 1984a).

Mrs. S's second picture (Picture 2), a watercolor, also involves pairs: two dogs and two suns (or the sun and the moon). The patient gives as her

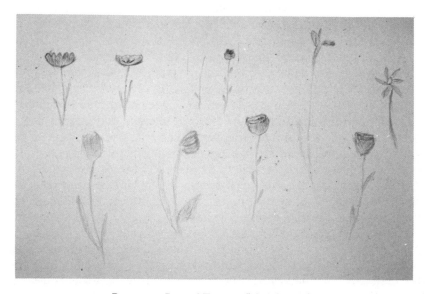

Picture 1. *Pairs of Flowers.* Colored pencils.

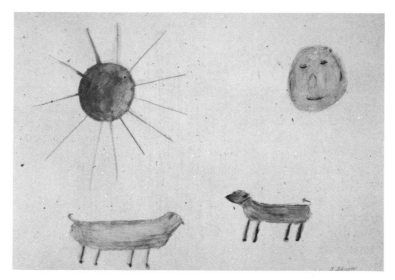

Picture 2. *Two Pairs.* Colored water pencils.

associations to it her grandmother and a little dog she had as a child, both of whom used to comfort her when she was ill. Already in the second session transference is beginning (the dog might represent a transitional object while the caring grandmother may be associated with the therapist). Again, as in the first picture, one of the two dogs seems less strong.

In the next picture (not shown), the patient depicted a dream she had immediately after being hospitalized. Owing to overcrowding at the university hospital, the patient spent her first night in a small auxiliary examination room. In the dream the patient found herself sitting in a ferris wheel while the people who sat above her kept kicking their feet into her back. Associated with the dream was her sense of being unappreciated by her husband and grown sons and her feeling that she could prove her worth to the family only by working extra hard in the house and on her job. Sick in the hospital, she feared that she would be as overlooked as a patient (put in the small auxiliary room) as she was at home. She was also afraid that, unable to continue functioning as a housewife, she would lose even the lowly position she had created for herself by dint of her hard work.

In Picture 3, the patient depicts herself lying unprotected in an oversized hospital bed. She explained that she lately had had no visitors and feared that her family had already forgotten her. The dying flowers by her bedside reminded her of those which one of her sons had brought her

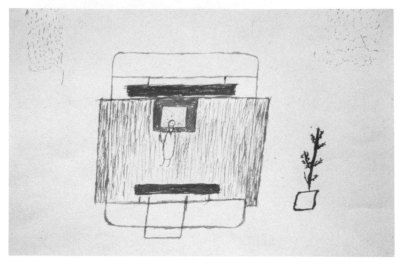

Picture 3. *I Am Lying in the Hospital Bed.* Colored markers.

on his last visit a week earlier; they symbolize her damaged, sick self, and the increase in her already strong sense of inferiority. She explained to the art therapist how she had drawn tears of sadness and disappointment on the pillow and in two corners of the picture.

This picture shows impressively how her leukemia provoked in the patient a fear of social isolation. It illustrates her denied rage against the malignant process and her uncaring family, and the depressive feelings that this denied rage caused. Through the medium of the picture, a transitional object that provided for this patient the basis for forging a secure relationship to the therapist, she was able to share her strong emotions and thus reduce the need to split them off. Recognizing the insecurity of her life allowed her to reintegrate her negative feelings into her personality.

Throughout her hospitalizations and during the periods of remission at home, Mrs. S continued to draw and paint. Drawing in her beloved garden at home, she found a means of communicating to her family and doctors and nurses the problems she faced as a sick housewife. She told me that she had recently asked her son at home to show her how to draw perspective, and he had illustrated by drawing the village street that led to the local cemetery. She asked me what I thought of this peculiar choice. She was greatly relieved when I suggested that it showed her son's fear of her impending death. When, some time later, the patient offered to draw for me the plan of her village, she was amazed to see the large gravestone for herself that she had unconsciously placed in the churchyard.

Mrs. S took her sketchbook wherever she went. It kept her company and secured the relationship to the healthy, intact, and creative parts of herself as well as to her art therapist, much as the child's teddy bear secures his relationship to the absent mother. The pictures, like a teddy bear, helped her to control her overwhelming fear of separation and to mourn her impending losses.

CASE 2

The following pictures were drawn by a 48-year-old office worker, Mr. P, who had been readmitted to the hospital after a relapse of his leukemia. He was married and the father of two grown children. I had already worked with him during his first hospitalization.

Without reviewing his entire art therapy (see Dreifuss, 1986), I would like to discuss five pictures the patient created during the last months of his life. They all represent different paths to his end. During his first hospitalization, the patient had developed a close transferential relationship with me. In his first picture after his relapse (Picture 4) he portrays, as he explained it, the hospital to the left and a Swiss chalet to the right. Dominating the center of the picture are huge steps leading up to the sky, with a tiny bicycle drawn on the first step. The patient associated to the chalet memories of his dream house in the Alps, where he used to retreat to be with nature. The hospital façade, with him looking out through a window at a black tree, obviously stood for his current situation. The steps, he said, lead to a "colorful sky"; they obviously represented his attempt to deny the threat of death. The bicycle might be said to represent his wish to connect somehow the two worlds, hospital and chalet, which he strongly experienced as separate at the time.

The second picture (Picture 5) depicts two portholes in the body of a big ship. Looking out at the sea, one sees the blue water alive with fish and underwater flowers that look like blood cells. The two portholes are supported by two green wooden ship ladders leading up to the sky and two wooden posts also reaching to the sky. Again we are impressed by the frequency of the pairs we find in this picture—an implicit statement of the need to find a harmonious inner balance. The ship's name is Zukunft (Future). As in the first picture, the steps seemed to lead upward, implicitly toward death, while the colorful water, with its living substance, conveys a comforting feeling of being contained within the therapeutic alliance.

The next picture (Picture 6) was first sketched and then carefully

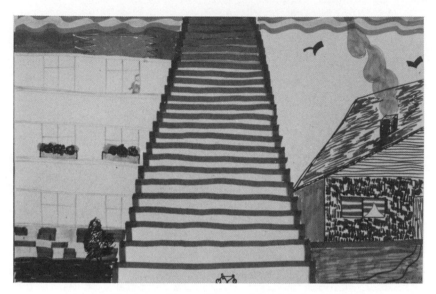

Picture 4. *Stairs to Heaven.* Colored markers.

colored in with water paints over two successive sessions. It contains two paths, which the patient explained come from opposite directions, that meet and lead to the church in the background, which is in the center of the village. The unified road then continues to the chalet (upper right) on a green field. The patient confided to me the joy he experienced when he used to go alone to "my Alp," where he felt supported by his farmer friends and in close touch with God and nature.

The next picture (Picture 7) shows the patient's awareness of the uncertainty of his future. Having been told by his oncologist that no further treatment was available to halt the malignant process, he and his very supportive wife had decided that he should go home for the time left. In the picture, he walks toward the sunset, the future, accompanied only by his own shadow, his double—signifying death. His shadow is projected in front; thus the patient departs in his picture from realism to find a personal, symbolic expression, better depicting his new sense of reality. As he left the session, he looked at the picture and commented that he did not feel alone, but supported and embedded in nature. The patient then asked me to continue his therapy at home.

On my first visit to his house, he asked me to start another drawing with him. He began to paint the "black curtain" that fell internally when he realized that he could no longer be treated after his leukemia had resisted

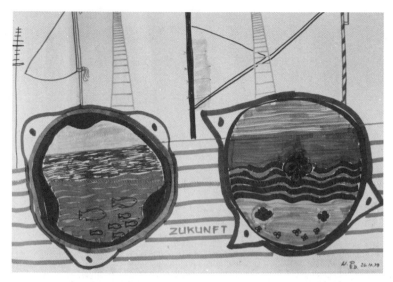

Picture 5. *Future*. Colored markers.

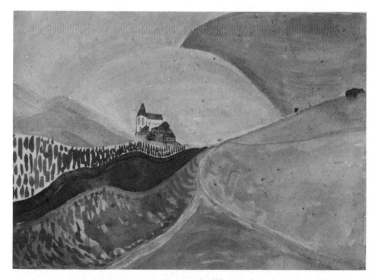

Picture 6. *Swiss Alp*. Watercolors.

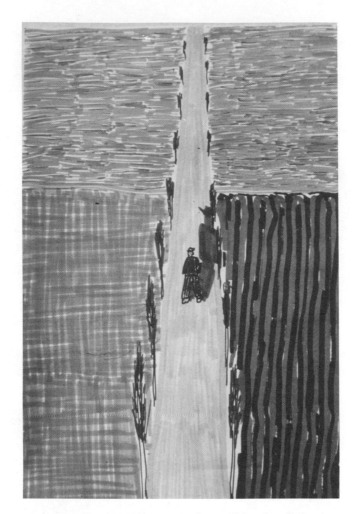

Picture 7.   *Walk Towards the Sunset.* Colored markers.

the most recent round of chemotherapy (Picture 8). He drew the curtain with a slit left open—a slit for hope, he said. He asked me to paint the foreground of the picture with various colors we had used together in the past—an indication that the sense of continuity provided by our sessions was still very important to him.

We worked for three more visits on the painting, and it seemed as though the patient was reluctant to finish this, his last creation. After an interruption of several days for Christmas vacation, on my next visit I found him much weaker and with a high fever. He could hardly eat. He

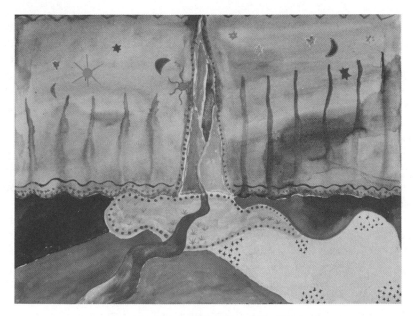

Picture 8. *The Curtain Is Not Closed Yet.* Watercolors.

said he was in torment because he kept seeing a vision that robbed him of his sleep. Since he was much too weak to draw it, he described the vision to me. It was of a very narrow path stretching out ahead of him. To the left and right was emptiness. The path led nowhere. Nothing was visible beyond the horizon. The stones with which the path was paved all looked the same. As I encouraged him to keep fantasizing about this vision, he realized how alone he felt on this narrow path. The interruption of the therapy for a few days had intensified his fear of death, and only my presence, which allowed him to share his fantasy, calmed the dying patient.

I reminded Mr. P of the many paths we had followed together over the past year in art therapy and how all of them had somehow been connected with nature. This induced him to talk about the good, secure, and even religious feelings he had had over the years in the shelter of nature. For the first time he told me how his father, who died when the patient was 16, used to take him hunting and hiking in the mountains and how comforting and exciting these trips had been. Stimulated by the therapeutic process and its transference relationship, the patient thus was able to retrieve the positive experiences of his past and recathect his good, internalized object (father). At the end of his life, the separation from his good internalized object thus seemed suspended.

CASE 3

The following three described pictures [not shown] were painted by a 38-year-old leukemia patient, Mrs. H. She was married, a housewife, and the mother of an 8-year-old son. In her first session, she verbalized her concern that her son might draw better than she, but by the end of the session she was proud of her first picture and hung it over her bed. In her next session, the patient told me how painting used to help her depressed husband, and she expressed her wish that art therapy would also help her now.

I worked with her from the first to the last cycle of her chemotherapy, about six months. Three pictures, drawn a few months into the therapy, illustrate a reactive regression following a temporary separation from the most important people caring for her.

In the first picture, painted just before Easter, the patient had fun playing with water and color and enjoyed being in good control of her brush strokes and the flow of color. After being rather closed in the period prior to the session she did this picture, the patient opened up to me and told me about the sorrows of the past year: her husband's heart attack and her little son's accident and operation. She told me of her fear of dealing with these hardships alone and unconsciously communicated her wish that I help her deal with her illness.

Toward the end of the session I reminded her of my coming Easter vacation, a three-day weekend. She immediately became downcast. This was to be her third separation. Her roommate, also a leukemia patient, with whom she had grown very close, had been allowed to leave for the holiday; and her doctor, whom she cared for very much, had recently left the hospital for good. Without thinking, I exacerbated her feeling of abandonment as I left by taking her pictures with me to show my supervisor.

At our next session after Easter, Mrs. H spontaneously painted a confused-looking picture, which, she explained, illustrated the fight of the good blood cells against the bad. She apologized for not being able to control the flow of water and color as well as she had previously been able to do. In discussing the picture, she spoke of her acute fear of the "strange" blood in her body (she had received a blood transfusion) and asked me how it would function in her body. The "strange blood" had increased the strong sense of estrangement Mrs. H already felt in the threatening environment of the hospital following the separation from her roommate, her doctor, and her therapist. The intensified feeling of strangeness led to a temporary loss of psychic control and motor coordination and, consequently, to fears of psychic and physical fragmentation.

At the next session, Mrs. H asked me whether I planned to stay in the hospital; she had heard that I was starting a private practice. I assured her that I would continue to work with her and other hospital patients. Thus reassured, she again began to take charge of herself, asking me for a form with which to draw a circle. I gave her a plate. She traced its outline as a starting point for a simple composition. She was content with her picture. The assurance I gave her of my presence (object constancy) after my absence, along with the technical assistance of an outside object (the plate), helped her to regain a sense of control after her regression. The elimination of the "strangeness" in the outside environment—my return was coupled with the appearance of a new physician—helped her to deal with her overwhelming fantasies of the internal strangeness due to the malignant process in her blood.

Without the confused picture of the good and bad blood cells, and the subsequent one of the plate, which enabled her first to dramatize and then to control her regression, it is likely that Mrs. H would simply have withdrawn into herself. The pictures enabled her to communicate her inner state without compelling her to recognize the intensity of her dependence on me. They provided her with the distance she needed to preserve her autonomy while they served as an instrument of communication.

CASE 4

Mrs. P, a 39-year-old widow, a school teacher, who lost her husband due to a motorcycle accident, requested art therapy when she suffered a second relapse of her acute leukemia and became aware of her impending death (see Dreifuss and Meerwein, 1984a). During her first interview the patient kept looking at my long hair. She told me that she too used to have long hair but had lost it through chemotherapy, which was why she was wearing a kerchief. Then she said that she had developed a compulsive need to look in the mirror, and she proceeded to take out a mirror and look at herself. It seemed as if the patient were confronting herself in me, in whom she saw her partly feared and partly wished for "double." It was as though she were saying, "I would like to be like you. I was once, but not any longer, which is why I have to keep checking in the mirror to see if it is true or not. In you I meet myself as not-me, in the mirror my not-me as myself" (Dreifuss and Meerwein, 1984).

At our second meeting Mrs. P spontaneously drew a little island with a palm tree. She commented that she still hoped to be able to find such an island, where she could save herself. When I asked her what she thought she might like to draw the next meeting, she answered, "I would like you to draw a second palm tree on this island." She thus unconsciously communicated her wish to find a companion, a double, in her threatening isolation. Before our next session she drew with the colored chalk I had left her a new picture, a strong, stable tree with empty branches, whose crown was mirrored in the form of underground roots, again suggesting mirroring a double underground.

In the next session, the patient told me that she had decided to return home, to another part of Switzerland, since no further treatment could be implemented. She drew two pictures, each containing a sad-looking woman, sitting. In one picture, the woman's hair was covered with a scarf; in the other, the black hair of the therapist was visible. The two women were waving goodbye to each other, the patient said. Shortly after her return home, Mrs. P died.

This very short relationship between patient and art therapist was dominated by the patient's strong wish to find an intact double so as not to be alone in her threatening isolation. This last relationship remained free of manifest conflicts and helped her to regain a certain rootedness, which eased her acceptance of death and made a real farewell possible.

Pairs are quite common in the pictures of leukemia patients. Since all the pictures discussed earlier were created within an art psychotherapeutic framework, we must understand these "doubles" in relation to the patient's object structure and especially with respect to its emergence in the transference relationship with the art therapist. The therapist unconsciously becomes for the patient a double (Dreifuss and Meerwein, 1984a). The leukemia patient most often sees in the therapist his healthy double, which he would like to introject so as to become narcissistically whole again. But at times, the mirror image, double, or shadow of a very sick patient can represent not only health and survival, but also the possibility of death, of the patient's not-being, and because of that it can become an object of great fear (Dreifuss and Meerwein, 1984).

The motif of the double is a recurrent one in Western literature and can be found in the works of Jean Paul, Kleist, E. T. A. Hoffman, Dostoyewski, Moerike, Poe, Rilke, and others. Its significance has been discussed by Rank (1914), Freud (1917b), Benedetti (1975), Dettmering (1978), and Dreifuss and Meerwein (1984a). Rank (1914) compared the double to the reflection Narcissus sees in the water. In the image of his double, Narcissus meets his own Ego. The double thus is really oneself, which one can simultaneously perceive from the outside: as I and not-I. The double thus has an intrinsically ambivalent character: the mirror image always reminds the subject of his possibly not being. The otherness of the double can stimulate anger as well as love and trigger a wish to destroy the double (v12. Oscar Wilde's *Dorian Gray*). By the same token, the loss of the double can also represent the threat of death. The superstitious belief that meeting one's double means approaching death can be understood in this context, as can the custom found in many cultures of covering the mirrors in a house where a dead body lies. Seeing one's image in the mirror in a house of mourning means dying. The shadow, reflection, and double all represent for Rank messengers of death.

Freud (1919) expanded on Rank's ideas:

> For the "double" was originally an insurance against the destruction of the ego, an "energetic denial of the power of death," as Rank says; and probably the 'immortal' soul was the first "double" of the body. This invention of doubling as a preservation against extinction has its counterpart in the language of dreams, which is fond of representing castration by a doubling or multiplication of a genital symbol. The same desire led the Ancient Egyptians to develop the art of making images of the dead in lasting materials. Such ideas, however, have sprung from the soil of unbounded self-love, from the primary narcissism which dominates the mind of the child and of primitive man. But when this stage has been surmounted, the "double" reverses its aspect. From having been an assurance of immortality, it becomes the uncanny harbinger of death.
>
> But it is not only this latter material, offensive as it is to the criticism of the ego, which may be incorporated in the idea of a double. There are also all the unfulfilled but possible futures to which we still like to cling in phantasy, all the striving of the ego which adverse external circumstances have crushed, and all our suppressed acts of volition which nourish in us the illusion. . . . [pp.235-236].

Leukemia patients are all particularly sensitive to the "striving of the ego," which their illness has thwarted (Dreifuss and Meerwein, 1984a).

The clinical consequence of the search for the double is the strong tendency of the leukemia patient to identify totally with his roommate, physician, or some significant member of the treatment team. That identification can serve as a source of strength and support in the patient's struggle with death, but it may also threaten his self-control, ego boundaries, and sense of independence and can result in a malignant regression. Then again, if the patient does not find a satisfactory "double" to introject, he may be left with only the experience of strong, repressed envy and consequent fears of retaliation by the envied person. As a result, a kind of negative doubling process occurs. To flee from this uncanny, dangerous rival, the leukemia patient may withdraw from and decathect his outside world.

The introduction of a transitional object in the form of a work of art or writing provides the leukemia patient with a safe stage and projection screen for his "doubling needs" and gives him an acceptable defense both against total fusion with the object and against a fantasied destruction of the envied surviving double, partly perceived in the therapist.

ART THERAPY WITH PATIENTS SUFFERING FROM A SOLID TUMOR

Unlike the leukemia patient, the tumor patient can localize his tumor in one or more ascertainable regions within his body. Thus, psychologically speaking, he can establish an internal connection between his tumor and the negative, dangerous, bad, threatening parts of his personality and can ward them off with the help of psychological defenses such as denial and projection. As a result, his sense of self is more stable and less threatened by fragmentation than that of the leukemia patient. The tumor patient is thus better prepared to enter into a relationship with the art therapist, who he hopes will help him to disclose the intact, healthy parts of his self and thus bring about a healing of the narcissistic lesion caused by the cancer. Owing to the greater amount of available psychic energy the tumor patient has, he is more ready than the leukemia patient to perceive the therapist as an independent personality and to form an attachment to him on that basis. This attachment promotes ready transference reactions involving both love and hate. The picture created within the art therapeutic relationship is for the tumor patient a direct tool in maintaining and developing a close relationship to the therapist, in whom the patient can confide and with whom he can compete in terms of exhibiting competence or even talent in executing the art work.

CASE 5

Mrs. L is a 39-year-old attractive, professional woman, twice divorced and the mother of two teenage sons. Two years after a mastectomy, she developed a metastasis that spread to her vertebrae and left her paralyzed from the waist down.

The therapy lasted for eight months.The patient drew a picture in each session, but here I will discuss only a few. The patient was outspoken, complained to nurses and doctors, but was well liked because of her direct, open way. (For further comments on this case, see Dreifuss-Kattan, 1986.) The first picture (Picture 9), drawn in our third session, illustrates what the patient said was a "vision" she had had. As she

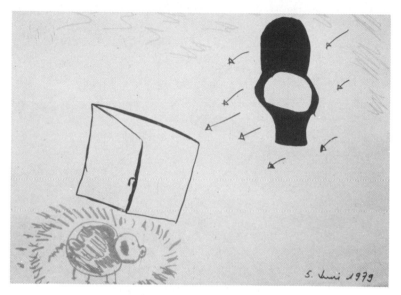

Picture 9. *A Vision.* Colored markers.

told it, a toilet bowl flying through her window turned into a lucky golden pig just before it reached her head. In our discussion it became apparent that the patient's anal aggression, represented by the toilet, was transferentially directed toward the younger, healthy, envied woman therapist whom she wanted to push away. At the same time, the patient hoped that her therapy (like her aggression) would turn into something good and keep the therapist with her.

Following this session, and in the wake of her father's cancellation of a planned visit and in anticipation of a short separation from me, the patient began to draw pictures that portrayed her sick, dependent, isolated patient-self. These, in turn, yielded new images, graphically portrayed, of her dependency.

The next picture (Picture 10) of this series shows two simultaneous images. On the left side we see an embryolike form enclosing a cross and a Star of David and linked to a telephone receiver—keeping the connection to herself. On the right side we see a storm, in which the patient, as she told it, fears she is drowning. Inside the storm two united hearts are swimming away, she explained. The patient's wish to unite with the therapist is illustrated by the cross and the Star of David, representing respectively her religion and mine, as well as by the two hearts, which represent a wish for union in the face of the dreaded separation of death. The same strong transference feelings were evident in the patient's

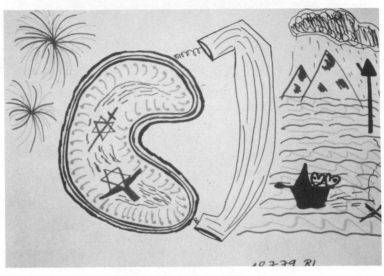

Picture 10. *Unions.* Colored markers.

conversation during the session. She explicitly expressed the wish to visit me at my home. Somewhat later, she went to town in a wheelchair cab and, through a series of missed turns, wound up on the street where she knew I lived. Around this time, too, she began talking of her hope that art therapy was putting her in touch with the creative, healthy part of herself. This hope was the subject of the following picture (Picture 11), drawn shortly before my vacation, which depicts a strong tree split in two. While autumn leaves hang limply on one side, new spring growth, representative of the creative energy stimulated·by the art therapeutic process, adorns the branches on the other. The patient feels she can let the therapist leave and yet continue to create.

The fourth picture (Picture 12), entitled "A Marriage Bell" by the patient, was drawn in my absence. It illustrates a close union between patient and therapist and between herself and her newly gained creative side. However, in contrast to the pictures by leukemia patients, where like objects are doubled, the two figures in this picture, a man and a woman, are distinctly different.

The fifth picture (Picture 13), showing a peacock, the symbol of immortality in Roman mythology, was stimulated by the resurgence of the patient's creative power. By its huge size, the peacock represents the eruption of a "phallic" defense (Hagglund, 1978) to which the patient now retreated. It is a magical force reinforcing her omnipotence despite her physical weakness and fear of death. The sixth picture (Picture 14) illustrates the other side of the strong defense: her awareness of the

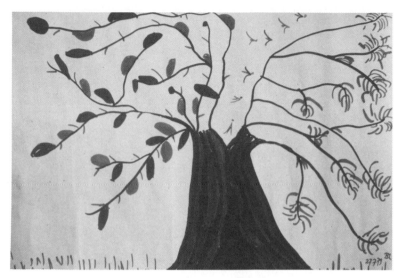

Picture 11. *The Split Tree.* Colored markers.

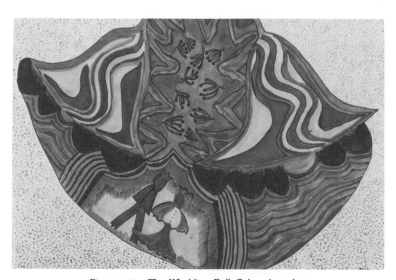

Picture 12. *The Wedding Bell.* Colored markers.

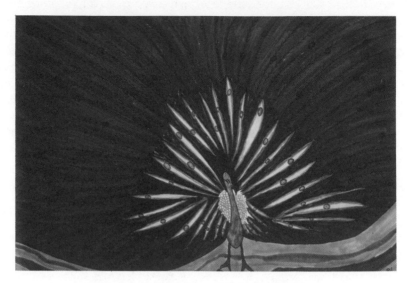

Picture 13.   *The Peacock.* Colored markers.

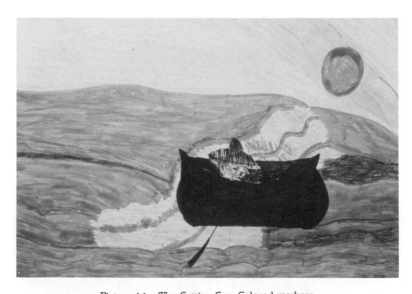

Picture 14.   *The Setting Sun.* Colored markers.

closeness of death. The coffinlike boat is moving toward the setting sun; its colors are mirrored in the patient's face.

Mrs. L could heal her damaged self-esteem through the positive experience of painting and through the relationship with her therapist. Her initial anal aggression, which previously had poured out on the treatment team, gradually transformed itself into a phallic defense, protecting her from overwhelming fear and loneliness. This defense also protected the patient from the envy and jealousy she felt toward the therapist and others who still possessed all those attributes she had lost during her illness. Painting was for Mrs. L a source of satisfaction and pleasure to the end of her life.

CASE 6

Ms. Z was a 42-year-old unmarried woman in the terminal stage of metastasized breast cancer (see Dreifuss and Meerwein, 1984a). As a result of radiation therapy for a metastasis in her lung, she suffered shortness of breath and was plagued by fears that she would suffocate. She was aware of her ultimately hopeless situation and realized that in spite of the experimental chemotherapy she was then being given, the terminal course of her illness could no longer be arrested. In the initial interview, as I explained the idea of art therapy to her, she volunteered that during the course of her hospitalizations she had often thought that if she could draw, she would paint a tiny worm being examined by a huge doctor.

The patient wanted to draw the first picture with me, so we worked on it together. The result was a picture of two nearly identical flowers in a vase that the patient drew. In this session, only our second meeting together, the patient and I already felt comfortable with one another. By the end of the session, her fear had diminished and her breathing had relaxed. In the next session Ms. Z was eager to start drawing on her own. She depicted a sky decorated with musical notes that also looked like cooking spoons, which she associated with the gourmet meals she cooked for her elderly father on weekends to win his favor. (The patient lived with her parents, and her mother insisted on doing all the cooking on weekdays.) She went on to draw a church while commenting that she was not really religious, then added two identical little flowers on the grass next to the church.

Suddenly the door of her hospital room opened and the new consulting oncologist entered, not realizing that a therapy session was taking place. Ignoring my request not to interrupt, he started to conduct a physical examination of her. Adding to her annoyance, he made jokes about the use of art in therapy and, in a critical tone, questioned me about its purpose. Irritated, I told him that I would explain another time. After the examination was over and he left the room, the patient started to cough badly. To the previously positive drawing, she now added a worm in the grass and, nearby, a little red ladybug. The unempathic intrusion of the oncology consultant had interrupted the initially positive working alliance, and the patient portrayed herself as the worm she had long fantasized—the helpless victim of the physician.

Moreover, the patient could no long regard the art therapist as a trusted companion. I was now represented in the image of the ladybug, a bringer of good luck, perhaps, but no protection against the intrusions of the doctor. The loss of confidence in my ability to guard the transitional "play" space resulted in a disturbing sense not of our mutual powerlessness, but of our differences. For unlike her, I could yet aspire to be the doctor's peer and thus become someone with whom the patient could no longer identify. As long as the patient had perceived me as a double, represented in the two nearly equal flowers in the first picture and the two little flowers in the churchyard in the second one, she could share with me her closeness to death, represented by the church she drew. The narcissistic injury inflicted by the unempathic doctor's intrusion made her feel like a worm again and emphasized the difference between herself and her therapist. Feelings of envy and jealousy of me were aroused, stemming in part from an early, unresolved oedipal conflict, which had been obliquely hinted at in her first picture of musical notes/cooking spoons. The same day, Ms. Z decided to go home with her old mother and she died there a few days later.

Initially, I suggested that the "double" is found in the works of leukemia patients, but not in those of tumor sufferers. In our last case, however, the same doubling process was evident in a terminal patient who suffered from metastasized breast cancer. Once the cancer spreads and the patient is in a physically regressed state, the cancer can no longer be localized and the threat of death becomes so overwhelming that it can foster the wish to find a double with whom to fuse so as not to approach death alone.

The reparative creative process that we see in these art therapy cases and in the literature of cancer patients helps them to reestablish the integrity of the self. Their creative products keep the integrity of the personality alive and help protect them from continuous fear, loneliness, and psychic disintegration. As 28-year-old cancer patient Dora Hauri (1982) writes:

> When I paint, I feel less pain. I am still aware of my approaching death, but it loses its tangibility; the thought is not

pointed any longer, nor is it blunt, it just exists. I feel that the
painting is inside me like a freshly sown plant and its fruit can
grow. With my paintings I can oppose my illness [p. 51].

The cancer patient is forced to mourn his body and the "objects" in
his external world. The losses are often replaced by various types of
fantasies, the most common being fantasies of immortality and of reunion
with a beloved dead family member or with Mother Earth. The losses can
also be replaced or compensated for by intensified relationships to the
patient's caretakers. Impending death leads many cancer patients to
reevaluate their lives. They review their experiences in the light of their
approaching death and make efforts to find a new, different wholeness.
Many cancer patients have a strong need to communicate their new
synthesis of their life experience to those close to them, whether
psychotherapist, doctor, or friend (Hagglund, 1978).

Fantasies are the cancer patient's last link to life. The loss of organized
fantasies that may result from the threat to life that cancer presents,
creates an unintegrated state and means total annihilation, utmost terror
and endless loneliness for the patient. On the other hand, creative work
keeps the patient from losing contact with his fantasies and counteracts
his fear of no longer being able to communicate his fantasies to those
close to him. Diggelmann (1979) demonstrates the importance of giving
creative expression to the pain and sorrow of losing an important person
or one's own physical integrity:

It was my only way, the only weapon I had to fight the
illness. So I arranged for this dictaphone 6 weeks ago. Because
I told myself, whatever happens to you, you're not going to
give up. You're going to change it. You're going to have to
make something out of it. You're going to have to use your
imagination. It's no use curling up and playing dead. You're
going to have to find new words for it. Words for my fear and
crying without simply saying I'm crying. They must encompass
my suffering and my physical pain without my saying I'm
hurting. A while ago, when they told me plainly what was
happening to me, a while ago I encountered death. He was
standing there, standing there outside my window. He begged
me to let him in; I did, I took him in [p. 102].

The patient confronted with his own death must gradually decathect
the outside world and cathect his internal world more strongly. In so doing
he internalizes whatever positive experiences he has had with external
objects and thus enhances his ego-feeling. In writing or painting, he shares

with others the fear and depression connected with the death threat. At the same time, his creative activity infuses his inner experiences with new life, a life that will survive his own. Freud (1914) writes, "What the artist aims at is to awake in us the same mental constellation as that which produced in him the impetus to create" (p. 212). For the cancer author or artist, this sharing is crucial, for it ratifies the inward creative response. "You're going to have to use your imagination. . . . You're going to have to find new words for it"—these words of Diggelmann (1979) are addressed equally to the reader. The joint imaginative adventure gives validity to the creative process and fosters a new sense of security that may help the patient to work through his fear of death or even overcome it.

Reading a book like Diggelmann's or contemplating a comparable picture, we identify with the strong feelings expressed by the artist/ patient. But at the same time we partake of the artist/patient's experience of form giving and internalization, that is, the recreation of the world that is being lost (Segal, 1952). We sense how the artist is dealing with his loss and transmitting the working-through process to us in such a way that the loss seems suspended. The reader or the art therapist identifies with the lost and rediscovered internal objects presented by the artist and integrates the associated fears and feelings into his own internal world through introjection. With the help of the cancer patient's book or work of art, the reader/therapist is able to establish contact with the artist who created it.

The content integrated by the therapist, if properly analyzed, may reveal not only the patient's immense sense of threat but also the dynamic structure of his inner world. This dynamic is embodied in his art works, in his pictures and stories. In art therapy, they make concrete symbolic exchange between patient and therapist. Within the art therapeutic treatment the therapist contains what has been put into her by the patient and so becomes the equivalent of a good mother who provides a safe space, a framework, and a medium where the patient threatened by death can move freely between the illusion of union and the fact of separateness, as happens in the transitional phase of infancy.

Within the context of the transference (or of a close friendship, as pointed out in chapter 11), the picture or story becomes a safe playground for the patient to exhibit his inner world and to alleviate separation anxiety, fear of loss, and fear of death.

13

Problems of Transference
and Countertransference
in Work with Cancer Patients

The ideal goal of psychoanalytic treatment is the development of the patient's ego functions. The patient should be freed of his infantile fixations, and the enhanced ego autonomy should lead to better inner and outer object relations. He should overcome his inner conflicts; his symptoms should disappear; and, at the end, a resolution of the transference and countertransference should mark a successful termination.

In the course of the psychoanalytic therapy of critically ill or dying cancer patients, an externalization of the ego functions becomes necessary; at the same time, external object relations are constantly reduced. Consequently, there cannot be a resolution of the transference which stands in great opposition to the ideals of psychoanalytically oriented psychotherapists, and it can activate a good deal of fear in the therapist. The death of a patient still strongly enmeshed in the transference can be felt to bring about a partial death in the therapist—and many therapists avoid it by refusing to enter into a therapeutic process in the first place.

Nevertheless, we do find individual case histories in the psychoanalytic literature that discuss the change of objection relations, the regression, the defense mechanisms, and the fantasy work characteristic of the terminally ill patient. The more extensive psychoanalytic studies are those of Eissler (1955), Hagglund (1978), and Norton (1963). It is interesting that all these cases involve cancer patients. This may be accounted for by several facts: 1) Cancer constitutes the second most prevalent cause of human death; 2) death by cancer is usually a slow process in which one can observe psychic development over a long period of time; 3) the malignant tumor often represents for the patient, both consciously and unconsciously, the bad part of his personality, or bad inner objects, and thereby directly influences the feelings of the patient's self and his relationships with others. The result is a great fear of annihilation and resulting isolation. The patient feels that his cancer intrudes from inside ("I am being eaten up by my cancer") so that the wish to enter psychotherapy includes thus the wish to empty his "psychic reality" of his bad introjects (Meerwein, 1987a)

The confrontation with death forces the cancer patient to undertake tremendous inner changes. On a narcissistic level, there is first the mourning of the lost integrity of his own body, which continually and painfully disintegrates. If we remember that the earliest development of the ego is closely connected with the image of an intact body ego, we can appreciate the threat to the feelings of self-worth that the patient experiences when his body disintegrates. Anger and shame are also brought on by the disintegration of the body. Most patients can withdraw the libidinal cathexis of their body and of most of the drive wishes and functions only by more strongly cathecting inner experiences and inner fantasies. Only then do they become capable of mourning the loss of the body. If a cancer patient cannot accomplish this change, he often becomes depressed.

On an object relations level, dying and mourning are also accompanied by a continuous withdrawal of cathexis from people and things in the outer world. The more ambivalent one's object relationships are, the greater are the difficulties that stand in the way of this withdrawal. In the terminal phase, the patient develops a strong wish to resolve the negative feelings toward his past and to the people closest to him and so to overcome this ambivalence. The better and more supportive these early internalized experiences stemming from the early mother-child relationship were, the easier it will be for the patient to mourn the loss of his outer world and to resolve his ambivalences. As well, dying people often try to give meaning to their lives by assuring their survival in the memory of their loved ones as good, loving human beings. They would like to be able to overcome feelings of guilt, anger, and envy and to be able to approach those close to them in a conflict-free way, leaving behind positive memories of their lives.

THE TRANSFERENCE FEELING OF THE PATIENT

The motive for initiating psychotherapy is often expressed by the cancer patient, frequently already in a progressed stage of his illness, as a statement to the effect that he feels he has lived wrongly. This can be heard as a statement that unconsciously he would like to regain and introject the "good" object that he has lost (by the emptying of his psychic reality) as a result of his cancer (Meerwein, 1987a).

As we stated earlier, the terminal patient is forced to mourn his body and the objects in his external world. The principal substitute for these—other than inner fantasies of immortality or of a reunion with a dead family member or of union with Mother Earth, and so on—consists of an intensified relationship to the people caring for him, primarily the psychotherapist. In forging that intensified relationship, the patient attempts to communicate to his psychotherapist a new synthesis of his life experience, one that is truly more representative of his present reality in the face of impending death (Hagglund, 1978).

In the initial stage of treatment, the therapist may become the recipient of transference from the patient's illness. The therapist can become the symbolic representation of the "cancer": he mistreats the patient by sadistically inflicting pain and suffering and otherwise conducts himself like a very bad internal object (Meerwein, 1987a). Part of the early work in therapy includes analyzing the patient's projections, first onto the therapist and then onto his cancer, and helping him distinguish clearly between them and the cancer itself (Searles, 1981). This clarification can bring the patient a great deal of relief. Once the therapeutic alliance is secured, both the life-threatened patient and the therapist experience intense giving and receiving.

For this reason, an idealized transference to the empathic therapist often develops, stemming from the patient's wish to regress to a very early condition of love, total security, and absolute trust. Handling the ambivalence that is inherent in any idealization is not easy. In the first phase of regression, one can see in some patients an externalization of the superego, or of its psychic antecedents such as the idealized parental image; this ambivalance image can seriously complicate the wish to identify with the therapist. The therapist, because of his youth, good health, vitality, or other qualities can quickly find himself in the role of the envied parent and can be rejected by the patient on the basis of the related negative affects of anger, disillusionment, envy, and rebellion. Rejecting the therapist often represents the only way for the patient to appease the harsh aspects of his superego as he attempts, by unilaterally ending the treatment, to ward off guilt feelings and fears of being rejected or abandoned.

Norton (1963) provides an impressive description of how one can interpret to the terminal patient these negative feelings of envy and jealousy in terms of the leftover conflicts from the oedipal phase. She interprets these feelings to the patient as an understandable replay of a childish reaction, which is reactivated because of the greater than usual dependence on the therapist and which ultimately constitutes a response to the malignant process of the illness. The patient's guilt may be relieved through this interpretation of the negative transference, and he will be able to reunite with the therapist and once more allow himself to entertain a wish for identification.

Another unconscious manifestation of oedipal envy has been observed by Searles (1981). He describes how the patient's cancer can be the point of departure for a "triangularization" of the therapeutic process. The patient can become a jealous rival in the triangle of patient, doctor, and tumor. The rivalry can be seen in patients who let their doctors (and therapists) know that they believe they are being treated only on account of the doctor's scientific interest in the tumor and not for their own sakes. The patient feels largely excluded and ignored; his cancer is the center of attention. Such envy is often overcome by reconstructing and working through the oedipal conflict.

In the second phase of regression, the therapist has to take over more and more of the patient's ego functions. She has to be ready to help the patient in certain daily activities that the patient can no longer manage. Norton (1963), for example, read to her patient as the patient became blind. This new, essentially maternal connection can help the patient to perceive the therapist as internally present, even when she is absent. As Norton (1963) says, "The borders between external and internal are at times hazy" (p. 555). Because of the internalization of the therapist, transference now becomes especially intense, something that Eissler (1973) believes is necessary. Eissler argues that through the intensification of the transference, the suffering of the patient, even when the pain is substantial, can be reduced to a minimum. With the transference, the therapist mobilizes an archaic trust in the world, which reawakens the essential feeling of mother's protection. Balint (1939) says, "The relation between mother and child is built upon the interdependence of the reciprocal instinctual aims" (p. 101) in which the love of the mother and the love for mother are felt to originate from the same source.

One feature of this primary partnership between therapist and patient is that it is always threatened by impending loss and thus has to be preserved at all times. Hence, it necessarily has an ambivalent character. This ambivalence has characteristics different from those of the oedipal rivalry. First, there is the wish to withdraw so as to anticipate separation; against this is the opposing wish to cling so as to avoid separation. Similarly, on the level of language and symbolic interchange, the immediate life threat also generates contrary wishes: to be told that everything is all right on one hand and for the illness to be taken seriously on the other. The following case vignettes illustrate the special problems of the cancer patient's transference.

CASE 1

Mrs. W, a 40-year-old shopowner, married and the mother of a 15-year-old boy and a five-year-old girl, had previously undergone a mastectomy for her breast cancer. Several years later she developed acute leukemia for which she was again hospitalized. Because of her great despair, art psychotherapy was indicated. However, the patient initially refused this offer, protesting that she simply could not draw. Her five-year-old daughter could do it better, she said, and would laugh at her when she saw what mommy had done. With this protest, the patient was expressing fear and shame over showing herself to the therapist as a breastless, childish, and underdeveloped woman. Her expectation was that if she drew poorly, the therapist would reject her just as her husband had threatened to do following her mastectomy. She did not want to expose herself to this threat a second time. After an interpretation, the patient settled down and was willing to work psychotherapeutically.

In the treatment, we worked through the feelings of envy under which the patient labored, which she had externalized by splitting her caretakers into good ones and bad ones. She perceived the nurses as bad and bossed them about, but she was friendly and compliant with her doctors. In the course of therapy, Mrs. W developed pneumonia and had intravenous tubes inserted in both arms and thus was forced into total motoric passivity. She became verbally aggressive toward the nurses and loudly expressed her feelings of envy, which made taking care of her very difficult. Unconsciously, she also tried to inactivate me by welcoming me back after a weekend with the words, "I thought you broke your leg skiing." She would frequently counter my therapeutic interventions with comments like, "You can talk well, you are pretty, young and healthy." Obviously such expressions of envy can evoke guilt feelings in the therapist. Against this, the therapist's unconscious identification with the patient, sometimes manifested in dreams, can resolve the guilt feelings. After the patient caught pneumonia, I dreamed that I was suffering from an incurable fungus infection of the lung.

In the course of her illness, Mrs. W was forced to go through yet another surgical intervention because of a relapse of her breast cancer. In the sessions following her surgery, the despairing patient recalled for the first time memories of her "good" grandmother, to whom she had been able to go in all sorts of difficult life situations from early childhood until adulthood. Her grandmother had nursed her when she was sick, protected her from her father's beatings, and favored her over her three sisters by singling her out for special little gifts. In comparison with this grandmother, her mother was perceived as "bad," without warmth, and unable to show her children love. However, at 65 the mother was still very healthy and, since her divorce from the father, was living with her boyfriend. "That, her living with a man, is why my mother is healthy," the terminally ill patient said enviously.

The interpretation of the split of both the nursing team and the therapist into a "good" grandmother and a "bad" mother, and the working through of the fear that her envy could destroy the "good" parts of the therapist, very much relieved the patient. She was then able to accept my help, internalize it, and so cathect her inner experiences more strongly. The loss of her sick, "bad" breast could be balanced out by the introjection of the "good" breast of the therapist, but that could take place only after her envy of the therapist's health, a derivative of the envy of the mother's health, had been worked through.

The intense relationship with the psychotherapist, who provides a "holding environment," can bring the patient hope, even in the face of impending death. We have to differentiate this hope from the initial denial that we encounter in the initial stage of the illness. If this initial "adaptive denial" persists to the terminal stage, then an inner sense of hopelessness develops silently in the patient and psychotherapy is contraindicated. The patient can express the hope by gaining access to primary process fantasies, which the patient experiences as a "freeing." "I live much more intensely than I did before," is a typical statement of patients in this stage. Control of the secondary process seems to be absent in this phase, and the patient tries to communicate to the therapist an "oceanic feeling." If this feeling is very strong, it can have a psychotic character and can confuse the patient's caretakers.

During the terminal phase, a distinctive splitting phenomenon often occurs in patients: the simultaneous realization of the closeness of death coupled with a belief that they will survive. The belief in continuing survival is often expressed in vivid fantasies of the future. Handling this half of the split is often very difficult for the therapist because it stands in such stark contrast to reality. The therapist has to accept this split and not try to obstruct it either by refusing to listen to the patient's fantasies or by denying the reality of the patient's impending death. As was pointed out in chapter 7, the therapist has to be able to sympathize with both parts of the patient, with the dying and the surviving selves. Only then can the therapist see to it that the patient feels held, supported, and accompanied to the end of his life as a whole human being (Dreifuss, 1986).

The next case vignette illustrates the regressive and intense transference reaction of a terminal patient in his last psychotherapy session.

CASE 2

I visited Z, a 24-year-old sarcoma patient at his home, where he had chosen to die. I had worked with him for nearly three years in art psychotherapy, accompanying him through numerous surgical, chemo-therapy, and radiotherapy treatments. For the past few days his room had been decorated with pictures he and I had painted in our art therapy sessions. Lung metastases prevented Z from breathing normally, and he was attached to an oxygen tank. He was feeling extremely weak; he was immobilized and could no longer sit up in bed without help.

As soon as I walked into his room, he immediately called me by name; it seems he was expecting my visit. In a soft voice, the patient told me, "I am dying. For the last few minutes I have been feeling this very strongly." Then he reached for my hand and held it tightly. "Your hand is nice and cool. Mine is very hot," he said holding on. Then he began to hum a waltz tune in a low voice and continued for several minutes. "This is a waltz," I commented. "Yes, I would love to dance a waltz now," he responded, his voice rising in excitement. I remained closely attentive but silent, not replying. Suddenly the patient started to beat his bedding with his hand, shattering the sense of peaceful intimacy that had grown in the few minutes. "It was all futile," he said, "my plans didn't work out. I wanted to live to my 25th birthday." Then he suddenly pulled back his covers and showed me his thin, sickly legs and his sexual organ. After that he asked me to replace his covers for him, which I did, feeling slightly insecure. "It was a good session," resumed Z, "when are you coming back?" He asked me to write the date of our next meeting (the next day) in his datebook, since he felt too weak to do it himself. He then thanked me for everything I had done for him and asked me to leave. Twenty-four hours later he was dead.

In this last session we both knew that he was very close to death, and the patient tried to use the session to anticipate his death through a kind of rehearsal. In his fantasy, he tried to fuse with me as a dance partner so as to attain the illusion that he would not have to dance his last dance alone. At the same time, he communicated a strong desire that I hold him close and protectively, like a baby, changing his diapers. In the gesture of uncovering his nakedness, he might have wanted to tell me, and himself, "We can no longer be one; we are not partners any more. I am terminally ill and dependent, and you are strong and healthy. We both have to accept this fact." It may have been his effort to provide me with a partial defense against the threat posed by a fusion with someone about to die.

The line between separation and union that the therapist and the patient both tread is a very fine one. The therapist must show some resistance toward the patient's desire for union. This is, however, not always easy. Sometimes one is forced to accept a parameter set by the patient. For example, in the case Norton (1963) describes, in a kind of symbolic realization of the fusion in death, the patient gave her a red dress to wear at her impending funeral. Norton agreed to accept and wear the garment.

In the view of Hagglund (1978), the most important task of therapists working with the terminally sick and dying is to bolster the patients' connections with their fantasy world, and to link the fantasies to the communication with the therapists. Fantasies, dreams, and transference affects all serve to bind the patient closer to the therapist; they help keep the patient's self coherent and prevent it from falling into an unintegrated state of terror and endless loneliness. Treatment of the dying patient must center around the so-called gift situation, as Eissler (1955/1973) called it. The crucial gift the therapist offers to the patient is that of himself as an available object (Norton, 1963).

THE COUNTERTRANSFERENCE OF THE THERAPIST

Because of the great personal challenge that the therapist accepts in working with the terminal patient, recognition and analysis of the countertransference are very important. As we stated in the introduction, the cancer patient who comes to psychotherapy would like to "empty his inner space" in order to get rid of his "bad" introjects, which, for him, represent his cancer. As a result, the patient feels empty while confronted with death. Clinically the patient's feelings come across as a "primary depression." The patient can say that he feels "I have lost my world," or, as Zorn (1977) puts it, that his cancer represents to him all the tears he has swallowed during his lifetime. In this situation, the therapist often feels that he is not in real contact with the patient. The therapist either identifies with the patient's empty internal space or else feels he is totally outside the patient's world. He may easily misinterpret the patient's emptiness as a secondary reaction to loss, castration, anxiety, anal rejection. Or the therapist may become easily overwhelmed by, and hopeless about, the immense task of dealing with this emptiness and as a result may refuse even to start psychotherapy with the cancer patient (Meerwein, 1987a).

Should they decide to establish a working alliance, the patient idealizes the therapist immediately. The therapist is now under pressure to "cure" the patient and can readily revive the therapist's sense of subjective omnipotence. Relapses and progressions of the malignancy, in the context of an overidentification with the patient, can easily leave the therapist depressed. Then, too, the patient threatened by death often exhibits ambivalent feelings: aggressive feelings on one hand, and wishes for union on the other.

Psychoanalytic authors describe the ambivalent character of the countertransference to the dying patient. The therapist's ambivalence stems from many sources. One is the mobilization of his own childish death wishes, which until now could be successfully defended against. These necessarily remind the therapist of his own mortality. Another is that the therapist knows that the end of the uncommon journey might well be the patient's death. If the patient dies, then the personality aspect that the therapist gave over to the patient will die with him. At the end of the journey, the therapist will not have the satisfaction of having helped the patient to a better autonomy and more mature object relations. In the end, there is a loss, which the therapist also has to mourn.

The therapist, as we saw in the previous example, is also confronted with his own guilt feelings that he will survive. His guilt and the patient's envy, sometimes even hatred, can burden him considerably. The result might be a heightened need to identify with the patient as a defense against guilt for surviving. But increased identification brings its own pitfalls and tends to mobilize various distancing mechanisms. These defenses, stimulated in the countertransference, can be expressed in various ways. The therapist might start to miss sessions or try to calm the patient with superficial comments. He might become overprotective or suddenly begin to overintellectualize the therapeutic dialogue. Such unconscious defenses aim at overcoming the ambivalence the therapist feels toward merging with the terminally ill patient.

These feelings of ambivalence, however, cannot be worked through, for they are inherent in working with cancer and other terminally ill patients (Dreifuss, 1986). The therapist must, instead, become aware of them and understand them. Only then can the therapist understand and help the patient. This can be seen in the following case vignette.

CASE 3

Thirty-seven years old and the mother of a five-year-old girl, Mrs. Y had to undergo a bone marrow transplantation after a relapse of her acute myelitic leukemia. The intervention was unsuccessful, and she eventually died after much suffering. The nursing team had cared for her intensively and was very highly motivated to try to relieve her intense suffering, which was partially caused by the treatment. At a team conference during the patient's terminal phase a nurse related a dream that the patient had conveyed to her. The patient dreamed that she was followed by hunters who hunted humans. She had to run away from them and was relieved to see, at the end of the dream, that a man was being saved. The dream made it clear to the nursing team how difficult it was for them to be put in the position of man-hunters who inflict pain and suffering on the patient, a position made all the worse by the fact that in the end, not the patient but someone else would survive the ordeal.

The dilemma of the nurses was conveyed in dreams that two nurses subsequently told to the patient's psychotherapist. One nurse dreamed that her grandmother was showing her the dead but beautiful patient and was pointing out to her how calm the patient now was. Another nurse dreamed that the patient had died but had to be hidden so that nobody would find her. Both nurses could hardly bear the suffering of the young patient, who, as a result of treatment, had become grossly deformed. Both to shorten the patient's suffering and to be freed from the position of hunters, they understandably had death wishes toward the patient and as a result felt ashamed and guilty. Fearing that the patient could read their death wishes on their faces, both nurses were afraid to enter the patient's room after having dreamed these dreams. The verbalization of these wishes and their acceptance by the patient's psychotherapist relieved the nurses considerably.

The therapist can also develop feelings of envy toward the patient, since, in a sense, the patient is ahead of the therapist in life experience. The patient "knows" more about when, and of what, he or she will die than the therapist does. The therapist can envy this knowledge and may need to defend against it by feeling guilty for surviving (Meerwein, 1987a).

In the terminal phase of treatment, we observe in the countertransference a feeling of being drawn into the dying process, as literally and figuratively the patient looks deeply into the therapist's eyes in search of a companion for this last journey. The danger of total identification with the patient in this phase can be counteracted only by a constant readiness to force a fresh triangulation through interpretation. This is the precondition for the establishment of hope and for the internalization by the patient of the "holding" that is represented by the therapist. Psychotherapists who work with dying cancer patients who cannot make the distinction between identification and interpretation will stand in the way of appropriate mourning work with their patients and deprive them of the hope of internalizing the "holding." Such therapists are always in danger of fusing with their patient in a primary-process hallucination of immortality.

For art psychotherapists, one avenue of detecting countertransference feelings is by way of art of their own creation. The process of self-observation through painting is similar to the so-called free floating attention that therapists bring to the therapeutic endeavor. The picture integrates primary and secondary processes and facilitates therapists' intuitive understanding of both transference and countertransference feelings.

I worked for nearly three years with Ms. B, an unmarried 42-year-old woman who worked for a publishing company. She had been suffering from breast cancer for five years and had undergone numerous operations and difficult chemotherapy and radiation treatments. We had established an excellent rapport, with the frequency and nature of our sessions altering with the state of her illness. Ms. B was not much older than I, also single, and had an interesting job and similar hobbies. She did not know of these similarities, however, since I tried to keep a neutral, therapeutic stance, even when she tried to coax me into a more personal one. With the help of the art therapy, the patient found a different means of expressing herself, as her old wish to write reasserted itself close to the end of her life. She was thankful to me for having helped her to attain this goal. Yet she also envied me my professional position and my independence and autonomy. Given our many similarities, I could all too easily identify with her. The more ill the patient became, the closer and, at the same time, the more ambivalent, our relationship grew. On one hand, I represented to the patient the healthy and creative parts of her own personality. But, on the other hand, I was also a mirror through which she saw the limitations of her life and her forthcoming death. Even though she attained some success with her literary publications, she increasingly realized that her creativity could not halt the malignant process of her illness, as she unconsciously hoped.

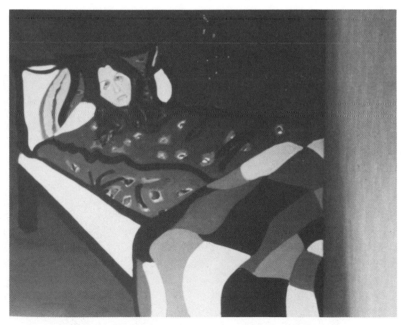

Picture 1. *Mrs. B in Bed*. Acrylic on canvas, 1 × 1 meter. Esther Dreifuss-Kattan. Verlag Hans Huber, Bern, 1986.

Supplementing intensive psychoanalytic supervision, I started to paint Ms. B in my free time at home, out of a strong, personal need. When I started to paint, the patient was already in the terminal phase of her illness and I visited her at home. In the first picture (Picture 1), I painted the patient realistically, lying in her bed. Her imploring look might be saying, "Come, do something for me." Both her position and her expression reflected her actual conduct. Whenever I arrived, the patient was happy to see me, eager to share her writing with me, but at the same time quick to communicate her frustration that whatever I had to give her was not enough. She wanted more, maybe my healthy body and my unlimited future. The red wooden toy that hung over her sickbed was transformed in my painting into a red cancer.

In Picture 2, I emphasized the more seductive, provocative quality of the patient. She fights flirtatiously with death, who is trying to push her down. As I looked at this picture, I came to realize for the first time that I strongly felt her trying to draw me in, to seduce me with an invitation to death, as though she were saying, "See, it's not all that bad, just join me."

In Picture 3, my wish for distancing manifests itself, as is clear from the perspective I drew. The patient now lies alone in her bed and seems to be hiding something under her blanket. In our sessions, Ms. B was

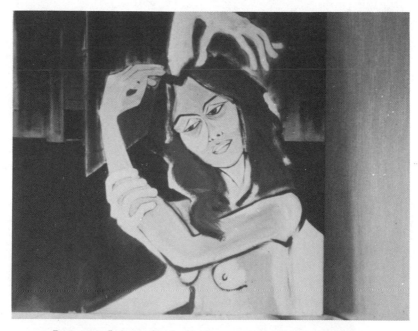

Picture 2. *Seducing Death.* Acrylic on canvas, 1 × 1 meter. Esther Dreifuss-Kattan. Verlag Hans Huber, Bern, 1986.

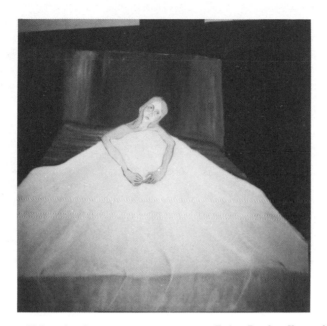

Picture 3. *Hiding.* Acrylic on canvas, 1 × 1 meter. Esther Dreifuss-Kattan. Verlag
Hans Huber, Bern, 1986.

beginning to talk more and more about her wish to commit suicide and
openly asked me to help her. I interpreted her suicidal wishes as a desire
to take her fate into her own hands, to regain control over her life and
destiny. At the same time I told her that I could not be of any assistance
in this act. Our visits became more and more difficult, and I felt clearly how
she wanted to draw me into her suicidal intentions. The pressure that I felt
must have inspired my fourth and last picture (Picture 4). In a virtual rage,
I painted eight hours straight, putting color over color in an all-day battle
on a two-meter canvas. Then I was utterly amazed at the result. There I
am sitting on the patient's stiff, dead body—as a corpse myself, identified
with her. I realized how eager I was to have this patient pass away, to be
done with her coaxing and cajoling, with her intense suffering and with her
longing to die, which had made me feel so guilty. I also felt guilty about all
the unexpressed hostility and anger that I had been accumulating and
about the death wish I had been harboring. I felt so guilty that, as I had
turned her into a corpse before her time, I transformed myself into a
corpse as well. It was as though I felt that only by dying myself could I
attain a guilt-free peace of mind after our long and painful encounter.

I had to act out my own death wishes on a creative level before I
could accompany Ms. B to the end of her life without aggression. I
realized my ambivalence only in my pictures. They enabled me to gain

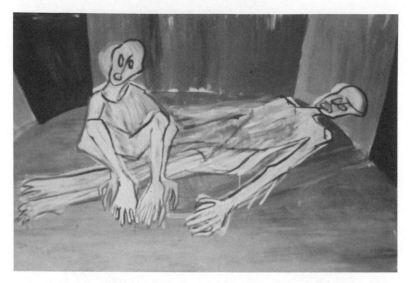

Picture 4. *Death.* Acrylic on canvas, 1 × 2 meter. Esther Dreifuss-Kattan. Verlag Hans Huber, Bern, 1986.

control over my ambivalence without mobilizing unconscious defenses in complete opposition to my understanding of the therapeutic process. Only if the psychotherapist can experience his feelings of hate as well as his feelings of love can he deal with his grief for the patient he has come to care for so deeply.

14

OBJECT LOSS
AND ART—
THE CANCER PATIENT'S FAMILY

In this chapter I describe several aspects of the mourning process as it surfaces in the bereavement work of the families of those who die of cancer. I illustrate the grieving process by examining the remarkable series of paintings by the Swiss artist Ferdinand Hodler in commemoration of his terminally ill mistress. I supplement the discussion of Hodler with material taken from art psychotherapy, where the process of mourning can also be seen in the content, form, and techniques used in the pictures drawn by surviving family members of cancer patients. We can consider mourning work successful when, following the mourning period, the bereaved person once again feels free to establish new relationships, to experience pleasure, and to reinvest his or her energies in satisfying endeavors and other forms of sublimation.

It is interesting that Freud, whose father died in 1897, attributed the creation of his classic *The Interpretation of Dreams* (1900) to his active mourning work for his father. Freud writes,

> For this book has a further subjective significance for me personally—a significance which I only grasped after I had completed it. It was, I found, a portion of my own self-analysis, my reaction to my father's death—that is to say, to the most important event, the most poignant loss, of a man's life [p. 25].

For Freud, as for Hodler, the successful completion of mourning resulted in an outstanding, enduring creation and a full, meaningful life thereafter.

FERDINAND HODLER: EXPRESSING LOVE BY PAINTING DEATH

I would like to introduce this subject with a series of pictures made by Hodler, between 1905 and 1915. Hodler drew, painted, and sculpted his model and lover Valentine Gode-Darel as she changed from a beautiful woman to a sick patient suffering and eventually dying from breast cancer. In over 50 oil paintings, 130 drawings, 200 sketches, and one piece of sculpture, Hodler illustrated how he perceived his lover "move from the vertical of life to the horizontal of death" (Kraft, 1984, p. 312). Hodler's pictures not only record the transformation of a sick person, but also illustrate how Hodler was able to live with Valentine's slow dying and at the same time overcome it through his art (Dreifuss, 1982).

An unconscious motive for Hodler's active artistic involvement in Valentine's dying might have been that his childhood was paved with many losses. When he was five years old he lost his father to tuberculosis. At 14 he had to carry his dead mother in from the pasture of their farm. Between six and 31 years old, he lost five brothers, his only sister, and a half-brother to tuberculosis, which was the major life-threatening illness of that time just as cancer is today. "In the family there was a constant dying, I felt as if there was always someone dead in our house and as if that's how it had to be" Hodler later recalled (Kraft, 1984, p. 318). When Hodler was 55, and in his second marriage, he met Valentine. Five years later she had a daughter by him. By that time, Valentine already had the breast cancer of which she was to die two years later.

Hodler's life shows a tragic chain of losses of beloved persons that early forced him to become preoccupied with mourning. His meaningful relationships were all very fragile and unreliable, in particular the one to his lover, Valentine. His only reliable partner seems to have been his art. His relationship to Valentine was tense, and as Kraft (1984) put it, "not poor of aggression, confrontation and guilt feelings" (p. 316) They separated often, only to be reunited again. He never divorced his second wife, not even after Valentine gave birth to his daughter. But Hodler visited her after she got sick. That periodic separations continued during the active phase of Valentine's illness shows the extent to which the relationship was marked by conflicts, fear of death, and guilt feelings.

With this cycle of pictures (see Nos. 1-6), the artist was able to work through the feelings of love, aggression, and guilt that are part of every mourning process. He not only portrayed Valentine's end, but captured death and dying as well. He created immortal works that have survived Valentine and the artist himself. His hope of regaining his once loved and now lost inner objects is illustrated in his fantasy of death: "When we think of Death, there is total unity," he wrote in his diary (in Kraft, 1984, p. 313). Through his painting, Hodler succeeded in regaining closeness to his dying lover and, at the same time, emotionally reviving his many childhood losses. While painting, he could process Valentine's dying and reintegrate it and his early losses into his personality. He confronted death by painting it.

This cycle of pictures has no parallel in art history. It starts with (Picture 1) a tribute to the beauty of femininity—the famous painting "La Parisienne" (1909) is but one example, for which Valentine stood model. In 1913 he celebrated the birth of their daughter in several drawings. Other pictures of that year, however, show us the first signs of Valentine's carcinoma. In 1914 Valentine had to be operated on. Before the operation, Hodler made his only sculpture of her, as though he needed to create her with his hands before allowing her to go under the surgeon's knife. Some months later, she had to be operated on again, and the pictures that follow (Pictures 2-6) illustrate the slow decay of the beautiful woman. By the end of 1914, there was no longer any hope for recovery, and the artist portrays Valentine lying back on her pillow, covered and with her eyes closed (Picture 4). In January of 1915, Valentine died and the artist painted the dead body three times (see Picture 5). He noted in his diary at this time,

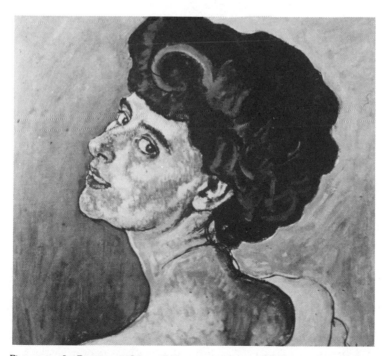

Picture 1. *La Parisienne*. Oil on Canvas, 41.5 cm. × 40.5 cm. Ferdinand Hodler, 1909. Private collection: Mrs. Lotti-Jenny-Zurlinden. Davos, Switzerland.

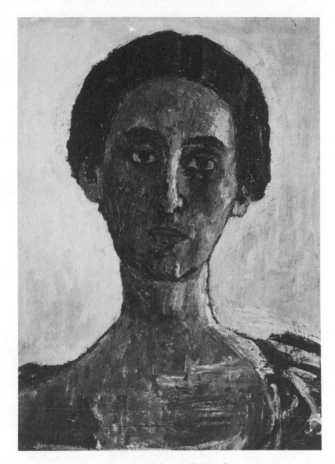

Picture 2.   *Portrait of Valentine Gode-Darel.* Oil on Canvas, 44.5 cm. × 35.5 cm.
Ferdinand Hodler, 1914. Private collection.

Death is the permanence of motionlessness, the absolute
unmoveableness of language. The permanence of nonlife is so
impressive because the observer realizes that he himself and
all others will also have to go there. All have to go there. We
must never forget that our similarity is greater than our
difference. . . [Kraft, 1984, p. 313].

Hodler's desperate efforts to recreate his lost inner object in his art is
also attested to by the fact that he often felt that his pictures were not
good enough, not concrete enough, not real. That is why he felt compelled
to sculpt Valentine before her mastectomy. Kraft (1984) quotes the artist:

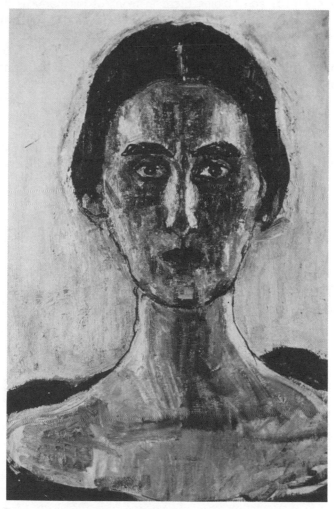

Picture 3. *Portrait of the Sick Valentine Gode-Darel.* Oil on Canvas, 148 cm. × 38
cm. Ferdinand Hodler, 1914. Private collection.

This beautiful head, this whole figure, . . . this nose, mouth—
the eyes, beautiful eyes—all this the worms will eat! Nothing of
it will remain, nothing at all! Or this stuff here? (pointing
off-handedly at his pictures), Just shreds, smeared and dirty
rags! Can one grasp them with one's hands? Can one take
these rags and shreds into one's arms? Can one hug them?
[p. 320].

"Thereupon, Hodler screamed with a pain-filled face, waving his hands in front of my eyes and holding them in front of his body as if to hug somebody," Kraft tells us. After January of 1915, Hodler made no more pictures of Valentine. We can assume that he had succeeded in working through his loss by that time.

Hodler's pictures reflect his mourning for his lover Valentine Gode-Darel and, at the same time, for the many dead family members and his lost inner object. His creating helped him to mourn the change and transformation of Valentine while she was dying and allowed him to express the various feelings her dying process evoked in him.

In the mid-80s, Hodler's picture series of Valentine's dying was exhibited in the Zurich Art Museum. They were seen by the Swiss artist

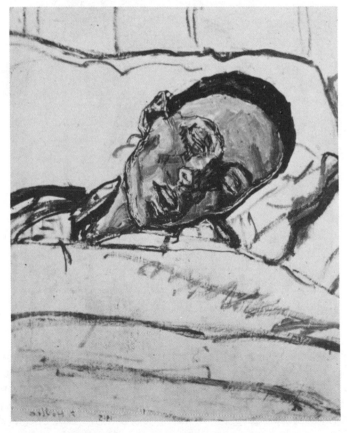

Picture 4. *The Dying Valentine Gode-Darel, Head Dropped to the Side.* Oil on Canvas, 53 cm. × 40 cm. Ferdinand Hodler, 1915. Private collection.

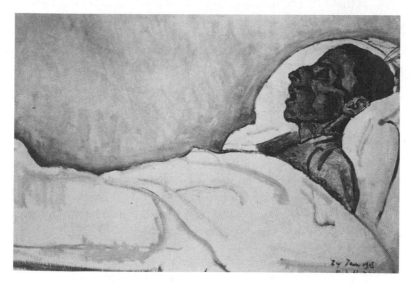

Picture 5. *The Dying Valentine Gode-Darel.* January 24, 1915. Ferdinand Hodler.
Public art collection, Basel Museum of Art.

and writer Erica Pedretti, who was herself then being treated for breast cancer. Inspired by the exhibition, Pedretti wrote the prize-winning novel, *Valery and the Ill-bred Eye* (1986). The novel features two main characters, Franz, who represents Ferdinand Hodler, and Valery, who represents his lover Valentine. Pedretti identifies herself alternately with the artist Franz, who paints his lover dying of cancer, and with the dying model Valery.

In the following passage, the author/patient tries to understand what the process of creating means both for the artist and for the patient, both for the healthy person who mourns his impending loss and for the one who is threatened by death. First, the passage where Pedretti (1986) identifies with Franz, (that is, Ferdinand Hodler):

> Feverishly he [Franz] draws what he recorded with one look when he entered. He draws it out of his head; he translates his fear to the paper, outside of himself. He draws this ailing invalid, her visible fear of death, out of his head where it continues to destroy, to slowly kill, so long as it is not somehow captured and made visible, and thus controllable. I have survived it once more, I still breathe, draw, draw my horror, my fear of death. . . . While drawing I am not afraid of anything other than my inability to record on paper what my eyes perceive.

In that I record the suffering, I distance myself. Clearly I am alive, I try hard, I work desperately on something which is not easy. To work concentratedly means for him [Franz] to live; concentrated it is not he [Franz] who dies, it is the other one who dies [pp. 148-149].

Then Pedretti identifies herself with Valery, that is, Valentine, Hodler's lover, who is dying of breast cancer:

Valery cannot take her eyes off Franz. It is as if each stroke of the pencil takes away a piece of her surface, her skin, piece by piece of her life. I am no longer what I was this morning. Without looking at the paper, I know that I am changing, that with every hour of his drawing my appearance becomes more and more remote. And he knows it too, and continues to draw. What kind of human being is it who has to record and make everything visible, so as not to be forever lost to him.

For him it is the picture. He does not want to deceive himself, nor does he want to deceive the observer. He wants to survive [p. 183].

To survive is what Hodler wanted.

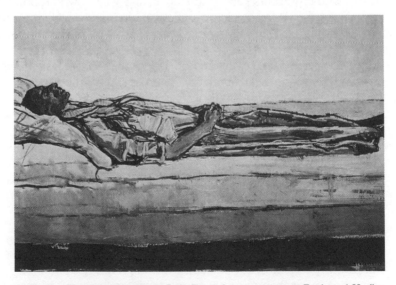

Picture 6. *The Dead Valentine Gode-Darel.* January 26, 1915. Ferdinand Hodler. Collection: Rudolph Staechelin Family Foundation, Basel.

ARTISTIC EXPRESSION AS AN AID IN THE WORKING THROUGH OF MOURNING FOR THE FAMILIES OF THOSE WHO HAVE DIED OF CANCER

The first reaction after learning of the death of a beloved person is shock and disbelief. The mourner's feelings are paralyzed and numbed, as aptly expressed in the talmudic image of the sword of death stuck between the mourner's shoulders (Dreifuss, 1983). Feelings of disbelief and strong identification with the dead dominate. At first, the sense of identification allows the mourner to deny the reality of the loss for a short period. Such denial through identification was exemplified by the lover of a woman I treated in the terminal stage of leukemia. After she died in his presence, he continued to hold on to her hand and refused to leave her room. I was summoned, and only after I led him out and interpreted his desire for union with his dead friend could he regain some distance from her.

Since anger and aggression toward the dead one are unthinkable at this time, the superego stands ready to retaliate for any expression of these feelings by evoking intense guilt feelings. The ambivalent feelings one naturally harbors for emotionally close persons include both love and hate, but in situations of mourning hate is taboo. Freud (1915) claimed that in the face of loss only the dreamer, the child, and the primitive allow their negative feelings to surface. Interestingly, many tribal death rites provide for an outlet of these aggressive feelings. They allow their mourners self-destructive acts, such as cutting themselves, which relieve them of their guilt feelings. In the Jewish religion, the *Keria*, the tearing of the mourner's clothes when a parent dies, symbolically expresses the same reaction. Therapeutic loss and mourning work can be successful only if the feelings of hate and aggression can be expressed and appropriately analyzed. If nothing counteracts the guilt feelings that arise from these negative urges and contribute to their continued suppression, a feeling of psychic immobilization can develop that will eventually turn into depression.

The following clinical case of art psychotherapy with a 42-year-old wife, who had lost her husband a year and a half earlier to melanoma, illustrates this point. (For further information, see Dreifuss, 1983.) She was referred to me because of depression, insomnia, and incipient abuse of alcohol, all consequences of inadequate mourning.

In her first collage (Picture 7), made from black and white pictures cut out of magazines, she shows us the beginning of a new year still dominated by the feeling of loss, symbolized by the empty armchair. In the second picture (Picture 8), also a collage, the patient illustrates how her depression keeps her imprisoned. The third picture (Picture 9)

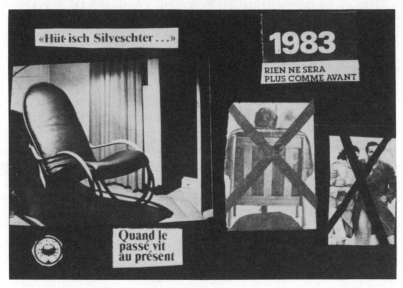

Picture 7.   *1983 – Nothing Will Be Any Longer as Before.* Black/white collage.

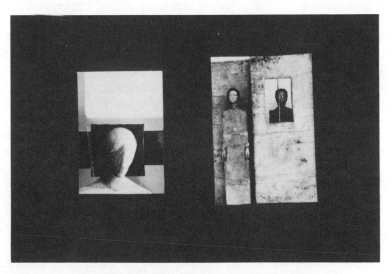

Picture 8.   *Depression Imprisoned.* Colored collage.

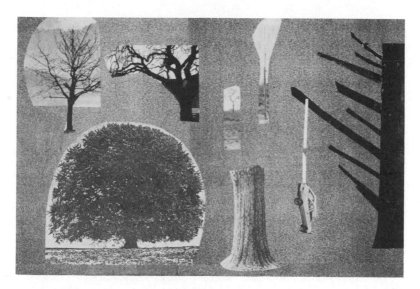

Picture 9. *Mourning Arrests Growth.* Collage and photocopy, black/white.

illustrates the contrast between the exuberant growth of spring that she perceived when her husband was alive and the arrest of growth after his death. The car in the picture conveys the wish to connect the two experiences.

As her sessions proceeded, Mrs. X realized how guilty she felt about the death of her husband. Till the last day of his illness he had insisted that she was responsible for his rapid decline, since she had pressured him to see a doctor. Her sense of guilt was expressed in a recurrent nightmare in which she saw her husband dead in his open coffin, his body badly mutilated as the result of an autopsy and was staring at her with reproachful eyes.

The fourth collage (Picture 10) illustrates Mrs. X's identification with the bad, dirty, aggressive cancer. The piece of paper reading, "The next one please!" (*Der naechste bitte!*), saved from a magazine, suggests that she is waiting to be caught by cancer as a punishment. At this time she also dreamed that she had a brain tumor, hardly surprising after all the time she had mentally heard her husband's accusations and had repressed her mounting anger toward him. The fifth picture (Picture 11) illustrates her mute repression and the wish that her head would explode and release its enormous pressure. The meaning of the sixth picture (Picture 12), a collage combining drawing and photocopy material, was clarified only by the patient's free associations. As a child, she had had no running water in her home and therefore was forced to shower at school. She was deeply ashamed of showering naked in front of the other girls, who showered at

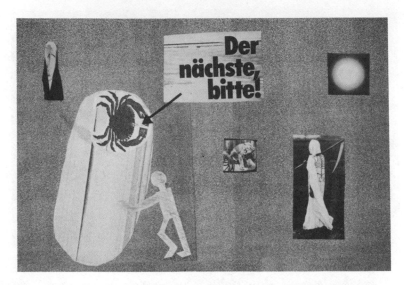

Picture 10. *The Next One Please.* Collage and photocopy, black/white.

home, and she envied them. Now in therapy, and feeling identified with
the dirty cancer, she hoped that her treatment would cleanse her and
make her like the other girls. The use of scissors in the technique of the
collage, incidentally, is also suggestive of her repressed anger toward her
dead husband.

The following quotation from Freud (1913c) captures the dynamics
underlying Mrs. X's strong guilt feelings:

> When a wife has lost her husband . . . it not infrequently
> happens that the survivor is overwhelmed by tormenting
> doubts . . . "obsessive self reproaches" as to whether she may
> not herself have been responsible for the death of this
> cherished being through some act of carelessness or neglect.
> No amount of recollection of the care she lavished on the
> sufferer, no amount of objective disproof of the accusation,
> serves to bring the torment to an end. It may be regarded as a
> pathological form of mourning, . . . We find that in a certain
> sense these obsessive self-reproaches are justified, and that
> this is why they are proof against contradictions and protests.
> It is not that the mourner was really responsible for the death
> or was really guilty of neglect, as the self-reproaches declare to
> be the case. None the less there was something in her—a wish
> that was unconscious to herself--which would not have been

dissatisfied by the occurrence of death and which might actually have brought it about if it had had the power [p. 60].

Latent aggressive feelings can stand in the way of proper mourning—as well as of creativity. The interrelationship of these two processes can be seen in the following case of a woman whose husband died of bronchial cancer. When her husband died, Mrs. B was the natural mother of their three children and the foster mother of a 14-year-old Asian girl. Between the Asian girl and the mother there had been intense competition for the man's love, and the mother often felt consciously envious of the adolescent girl, who was very beautiful. When the husband became ill, the girl left the house, returning only after her stepfather had died. Her move seems to have been motivated, at least in part, by fear of her envious stepmother's revenge.

In therapy, Mrs. B confronted her feelings that her aggression had contributed to her husband's death. The first face she painted in therapy amazed her with its angry expression; in an attempt not to acknowledge the feeling, she promptly covered the face with masking tape (Picture 13). The inhibition continued and somewhat later, when she was asked to draw from memory the face of someone in her therapy group, she could draw only the contours of the face, this despite years at art school (Picture 14). This second picture illustrated how her depression, which covered up her

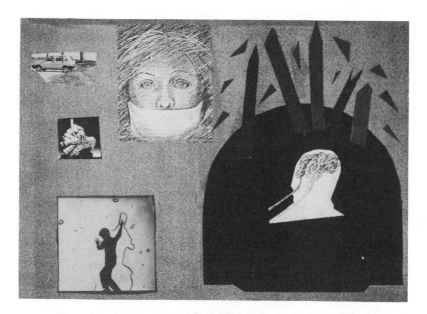

Picture 11. *Release of Tension.* Collage and photocopy, black/white.

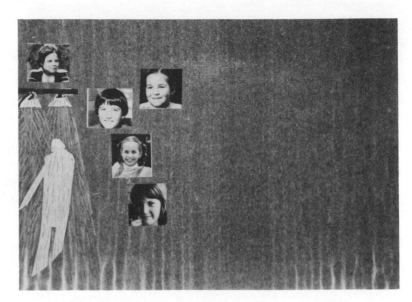

Picture 12. *The Shower.* Collage and photocopy, black/white.

anger, actually blocked her ability to perceive another person. It was less a drawing than the expression of an inhibition of drawing.

In the next session I asked the patient to make a picture of some place where she thought she would feel comfortable (Picture 15). For the first time, Mrs. B became involved. She chose to do a collage showing the head of a dead man in a wooden coffin topped by a big black cross. She placed a sad-faced picture of herself looking into the picture. This work represents her achievement of an aesthetic sense of distance from her anger, for which the scissors used in the collage technique had provided a motor outlet. Following this session she was able to draw and create as well as deal with the pain of her husband's death.

In the second phase of mourning, which is illustrated in the talmudic image of the sword placed in front of and pointed at the mourner (so that he can look at it), the mourner is forced to face the reality of the beloved person's absence. Pollock (1978) calls it the time for catharsis through talking, the time when the mourner finds relief in talking to his family and friends about the dead person. Sometimes, however, such talk does not so much help the mourner to come to terms with the death as it serves as a means of holding on to the dead person.

As Freud (1917) writes, although "mourning involves grave departures from the normal attitude to life, it never occurs to us to regard it as a pathological condition. . . . We rely on its being overcome after a certain

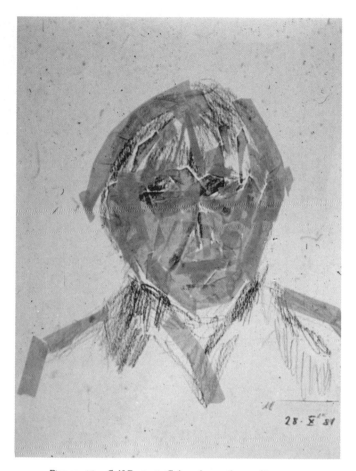

Picture 13. *Self-Portrait.* Colored pencils, masking tape.

lapse of time. . ." (pp. 243–244). Freud also makes note, however, of the "understandable opposition" against the withdrawal of the libido from the dead one. "This opposition," he says, "can be so intense that a turning away from reality takes place and a clinging to the object through the medium of a hallucinatory wishful psychosis" (p. 244). For example, the boyfriend of the leukemia patient who did not want to leave the room after her death, had a great deal of difficulty relinquishing his desire to be reunited with his dead friend; his strong initial denial of her death continued for a time in a fantasy of his dead girlfriend's having become a protecting angel that followed him everywhere. In this fantasy the separation brought about through death was suspended. At times the fantasy became very vivid, much like a hallucinatory wish fulfillment.

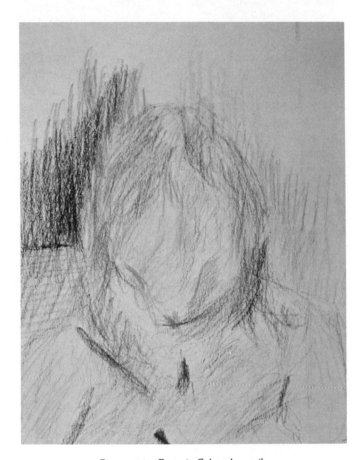

Picture 14. *Portrait.* Colored pencils.

Progressive mourning work, however, helped him to relinquish this fantasy and face the reality of life without his girlfriend.

Rumination about the dead is part of a normal process fostered in the consoler's visits to the bereaved. It can also turn into a pathological search, as it was for a 13-year-old boy referred for therapy by his mother when she was dying of breast cancer. The boy had been born with a physical disorder that made him unduly dependent on his mother. He had been kept so symbiotically dependent that when his mother was terminally ill, he declared, "When you die I will die too." After she died, he unconsciously feared that the strong aggressive feelings that his dependency

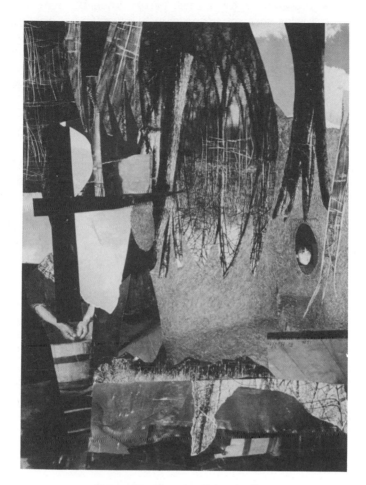

Picture 15. *Mourning.* Colored collage.

had fostered might have killed her. Subsequently he insisted that the therapist accompany him in a search for her in the dark basement rooms in the hospital where she had been treated.

The next phase of mourning is again illustrated in a talmudic image: the Sword of Death follows the mourner into the marketplace. Even though the mourner is still closely connected to his experience of loss, he now returns to work and rejoins the community. A full year, with its span of seasons, feelings, and memories reviving the pain of loss seems for many to be an appropriate length of time to complete mourning. This idea is illustrated by a young widow I treated, a mother of three small children. On her last birthday before his death, her terminally ill husband had helped her with the preparations for a small party. When her birthday came around the following year, she unconsciously expected her eight-year-old son to take the dead father's place in the birthday preparations. When, in therapy, she became aware of her excessive demands on her young son, she once again found herself mourning the loss of her husband.

Creativity can play an important role in coping with the loss and the mourning of a beloved person. In mourning, libido is withdrawn as a result of object loss; in creativity, a similar withdrawal occurs as a result of regression reflected in a longing for the illusion of the mother and child mutuality of the transitional phase. In writing or drawing the bereaved can find comfort for his or her loss by creating something new. The ambivalent feelings inherent in the loss of an important object can also be safely channeled into creative work; there they can be recognized and reintegrated and thus make their own contribution to redefining an inner organization. The art work assists the bereaved to establish a new narcissistic equilibrium. The dead object need not totally disappear emotionally; its memory can always be revived and memorialized in the work of art.

I would like to end with a quotation by Hodler (cited in Kraft, 1984):

That's how death approaches us, each second of our lives: it is a quiet movement and a counter-movement. If you take Death into your knowledge, into your will, you can create impressive works. You have only this one life to fulfill yourself. Death structures our entire life, providing it with a totally different rhythm. To accept it, transforms the death-thought into a powerful force [p. 322].

References

Alsop, S. (1973), *Stay of Execution*. Philadelphia: Lippincott.

Auchter, T. (1978), Die Suche nach Vorgestern, Trauer und Kreativitaet. *Psyche* 1:52-77.

Badruddin, K. (1982), *Poems of Gitanjali*. London: Oriel Press.

Baines, M. (1984), Cancer pain. *Postgrad. Med. J.*, 60:852-857.

Balint, A. (1939), Love for the mother and mother love. In: *Primary Love and Psychoanalytic Technique*, ed. M. Balint. New York: Liveright.

Baltrush, H. (1969), Psychosomatische Beziehungen bei Krebspatienten. *Psychosom. Med.* 15-31:196-215.

Benedetti, G. (1975), *Psychiatrische Aspekte des Schoepferischen*. Goettingen: Vandenhoeck & Ruprecht.

Beutler, M. (1980), *Fussfassen*. [*Settling Down*]. Bern: Zytglooge.

Bibring, G. (1961), The mechanism of depression. In: *Affective Disorders*, ed. P. Greenacre. New York: International Universities Press.

Brueschweiler, J. (1976), *Ferdinand Hodler: Ein Maler vor Liebe und Tod*. Zurich: Kunsthaus, Brueschweiler Jura.

Buchanan, W. (1978), *A Shining Season*. Albuquerque: University of New Mexico.

Cassileth, B. & Cassileth, P. (1982), *Clinical Care of the Terminal Cancer Patient*. Philadelphia, PA: Lea & Febiger.

Chasseguet-Smirgel, J. (1984a), Thought on the concept of reparation and the hierarchy of creative acts. *Internat. Rev. Psycho-Anal.*, 11:399-406.

_____ (1984b), *Creativity and Perversion*. London: Free Association Books.

Diggelmann, W. (1979), *Schatten Tagebuch einer Krankheit*. [*Shadows, Diary of an Illness*]. Zuerich: Benziger.

Dittmering, P. (1978), Doppelgaengererfahrung, In: *Dichtung und Psychoanalyse, Vol. 12*, ed. H. V. Doderer, Fachbuchhandlung Psychologie.

Dreifuss, E. (1982), Der Krebspatient und seine Familie — Erfahrungen aus der

245

Klinik. *Schweizerische Rundschau fur Medizin*, 49:1927-1934.

_____ (1983), Verlust und Trauerarbeit in der juedischen Tradition. *Schweizerisch Aerztezeitung*, 64(46):1928-1935.

_____ & Meerwein, F. (1984a), Das Doppelgaenger-motiv. *Zeitschrift fuer Psychosom. Med. und Psychoanal*, 3:282-291.

Dreifuss-Kattan, E. (1986), *Praxis der Klinischen Kunsttherapie*. Bern: Hans Huber.

_____ (1988), The psychotherapeutic significance of art therapy in the treatment of adult cancer patients. *Japanese Bull. Art Therapy*, 19:89-99.

Dreifuss-Kattan, E. & Meerwein, F. (1984b), Die Psychotherapie Sterbender-Der Beitrag der Psychoanalyse. In: *Die Begleitung Sterbender*, ed. I. Spiegel-Roesing, H. Petzold. Padeborn: Junfernmann.

Eissler, K. (1955), *The Psychiatrist and the Dying Patient*. New York: International Universities Press, 1973.

Fiore, N. (1979), Fighting cancer: One patient's perspective. *New Eng. J. Med.*, 300:284-289.

Freud, S. (1900), The interpretation of dreams. *Standard Edition*, 9:141-154. London: Hogarth Press, 1959.

_____ (1908), Creative writers and day-dreaming. *Standard Edition*, 9:141-154. London: Hogarth Press, 1959.

_____ (1909), Leonardo da Vinci, memories of his childhood. *Standard Edition*, 11:63-137. London: Hogarth Press, 1957.

_____ (1913a), The claims of psycho-analysis to scientific interest. *Standard Edition*, 13:165-189. London: Hogarth Press, 1953.

_____ (1913b), The theme of the three caskets. *Standard Edition*, 12:289-302, London: Hogarth Press, 1958.

_____ (1913c), Totem and taboo. *Standard Edition*, 13:1-161. London: Hogarth Press, 1953.

_____ (1914), The Moses of Michelangelo. *Standard Edition*, 13:211-236. London: Hogarth Press, 1958.

_____ (1915), Thoughts for the times on war and death. *Standard Edition*, 14:109-140, London: Hogarth Press, 1959.

_____ (1917), Mourning and melancholia. *Standard Edition*, 14:237-258, London: Hogarth Press, 1957.

_____ (1919), The uncanny. *Standard Edition*, 17:217-262, London: Hogarth Press, 1955.

_____ (1924a), An autobiographical study. *Standard Edition*, 20:7-39, London, Hogarth Press, 1959.

_____ (1924b), The resistances to psychoanalysis. *Standard Edition*, 19:213-222, London: Hogarth Press.

_____ (1926), Inhibitions, symptoms and anxiety. *Standard Edition*, 20:75-176, London: Hogarth Press, 1959.

_____ (1927), The future of an illusion. *Standard Edition*, 21:64-65, London: Hogarth Press, 1961.

_____ (1928), Dostoevsky and parricide. *Standard Edition*, 21:175-196, London: Hogarth Press, 1961.

Goldberg, G. (1981), Medicine as food: Exploring the unconscious meanings of cancer treatment. In: *Psychotherapeutic Treatment of Cancer Patients*, ed. G.

Goldberg. New York: Free Press.

Golub, S. (1981), Coping with cancer: Freud's experiences. *Psychoanal. Rev.,* 68:191-200.

Greenberger, E. (1965), Fantasies of a woman confronting death. *J. Consul. Psychol.,* 29:252-260.

Greer, S., Morris, T. & Pettingale, K. (1979), Psychological response to breast cancer: Effect on outcome. *Cancer,* 13:785-787.

Hackett, T., Cassem, N., & Raker, J. (1973), Patients' delay in cancer. *New Eng. J. Med.,* 289:14-20.

Haefliger, U. (1988), Versuch uner Entwicklungslinie des Zeiterlebens. Unpublished manuscript. Zuerich.

Hagglund, T. (1978), *Dying, A Psychoanalytic Study with Special References to Individual Creativity and Defense Organization.* New York: International Universities Press.

———— (1980), The dying patient. Lecture presented at the International Conference of Psychoanalysis, New York City.

Hauri, D. (1982), *Ich habe den Herbst gesehen* [*I Have Seen Fall*]. Basel: Mond-Buch.

Henze, C. (1987), Poems by Claire Henze. In: *Confronting Cancer Through Art,* ed. Regents of the University of California. Los Angeles: Jonsson Comprehensive Cancer Center at the University of California.

Higginbotham, M. (1974), *With Each Passing Moment.* Tampa, FL: Grace.

Hoffer, W. (1964), Mund, Hand und Ich-Integration; *Psyche,* 6:2.

Hosch, T. (1986), *Krebs Von Januar bis August? Stationen einer Morbus - Hodgkin Erkrankung.* [*Cancer from January to August? Stations of a Morbus Hodgkins Disease*]. Heidelberg: Verlag fuer Medizin.

Howe, H. (1981), *Do Not Go Gentle.* New York: Norton.

James, A. (1964), *The Diary of Alice James,* ed. L. Edel. New York: Dodd Mead.

Jones, E. (1957), *The Life and Work of Sigmund Freud,* Vol 3. New York: Basic Books.

Klein, M. (1948), *Contribution to Psycho-Analysis.* London: Hogarth Press.

———— (1975), *Envy and Gratitude.* New York: Delacorte Press.

———— (1975), *Love, Guilt and Reparation and Other Works 1921-1945.* New York: Delacorte Press.

Kohut, H. (1975), Kreativitaet, Charisma, Gruppenpsychologie, *Psyche,* 8:681-720.

Kovner, A. (1988a), Transparence. *Tel Aviv Review,* 1.

———— (1988b), In their infuriating confidence. *Tel Aviv Review,* 1.

Kraft, H. (1984), Objektverlust und Kreativitaet—eine Darstellung anhand Ferdinand Holder's Werkzyklus ueber Valentine Gode-Darel. In: *Psychoanalyse, Kunst und Kreativitaet,* ed. H. Kraft. Koeln: DuMont Buehverlag.

Kubler-Ross, E. (1969), *On Death and Dying.* New York: MacMillan.

Langer, C. (1989), The art of healing. *Ms. Magazine,* Jan./Feb., p. 132.

Langer, S. (1953) *Feeling and Form,* New York: Charles Scribner's Sons.

Lazarus, R. (1981), The costs and benefits of denial, In: *Stressful Life Events and Their Contexts, Monographs in Psychological Epidemiology,* Vol. 2, ed. B. Dohrenwend. New York: Watson.

Lenker, C. (1984), *Krebs Kann auch eine Chance Sein.* [*Cancer Can Also Be a*

Chance]. Frankfurt: Fischer Taschenbuch.

Lichtenberg, J. D. (1983), *Psychoanalysis and Infant Research*. Hillsdale, NJ: The Analytic Press.

Lipowski, Z. (1970), Physical illness, the individual and the coping process. *Psychiat. Med.* 1:91-102.

Lorde, A. (1980), *The Cancer Journals*. San Francisco: Spinsters/Aunt Lute.

Masson, J. ed. (1985), *The Complete Letters of Sigmund Freud to Wilhelm Fliess, 1887-1904*. Cambridge, MA: Harvard University Press.

Meerwein, F., ed. (1985a), *Einfuerhueng in die Psycho-onkologie*. Bern, Stuttgart, Toronto: Hans Huber.

_____ (1985b) Das Erstgespraech auf der Abteilung fuer Onkologie. In: *Das therapeutische Gespraech mit Krebs-patienten*, ed. W. Brautigam & F. Meerwein. Bern: Hans Huber.

_____ (1986a), *Das aerzlische Gespraech*. Bern: Hans Huber.

_____ (1986b), Selbstaggression, Selbstzerstoerung, Suizid in der psychosomatischen Medizin unter besonderer Beruecksichtigung der Krebskrankheiten. In: *Selbstaggression, Selbstzerstoerung, Suizid*, Band 6, ed. H. Braun & Zuercher Hochschulforum. Zurich: Artemis.

_____ (1987a), Bemerkungen zur Metapsychologie schwerer Krebserkrankungen. *Bulletin der Schweiz. Gesellschaft fuer Psychoanal.*, 32:123-196.

_____ (1987b), Angst vor Wahrheit am Krankenbett. In: *Angst*, ed. H. Schulz. Stuttgart: Kreutz.

_____ (1988), Cancer, symbolic representation of bad inner images. Unpublished manuscript.

_____ (1989), Zeiterleben im psychoanalytischen Prozess. *Psychosomatische Medizin u. Psychoanal.*, 2:156-174.

Meerwein, P. (1980), *Der Krebspatient und sein Arzt im 19 Jahrhundert*. Zurich: Juris.

Metzger, D. (1983), I am no longer afraid. In: *Tree*. Berkeley, CA: Wingbow Press.

Michie, M. (1980), A splendid day. *Virginia Quart. Rev.*, 56:410-423.

Mullan, F. (1985), *Vital Signs*. New York: Farrar, Straus & Giroux.

_____ (1987), A midwife to art. In: *Confronting Cancer Through Art*, ed. Regents of the University of California. Los Angeles: Jonsson Comprehensive Cancer Center at the University of California.

Murray, M. (1975), *The Great Mother and Other Poems*. New York: Sheed & Ward.

Muschg, A. (1981), *Literatur als Therapie?* Band 65. Frankfurt Suhrkamp.

Nelson, R. (1981), The final victory of General U.S. Grant. *Cancer*, 47:483-436.

Noll, P. (1984), *Diktate ueber Sterben und Tod*. [*Dictations on Death and Dying*]. Munich: Serie Piper.

Norton, J. (1963), Treatment of a dying patient. *The Psychoanalytic Study of the Child*, 25:360-400, New York: International Universities Press.

Pao, P. (1983), Suspension of the reality principle in adaptation and creativity. *Psychoanal. Inq.*, 3:431-449.

Pedretti, E. (1986), *Valerie oder das unerzogene Auge*. [*Valery of the Ill-bred Eye*]. Frankfurt: Suhrkamp.

Pietzeker, C. (1978), Zur Psychoanalyse der Literarischen Form., In: *Perspektiven Psychoanalytischer Literaturkritik*, ed. S. Goepperts. Freiburg: Rombach.

Pollock, G. (1978), Process and affect: Mourning and grief. *Internat. J. Psycho-Anal.*, 59:255-276.

Portenoy, R. & Foley, K. (1989), Management of cancer pain. In: *Handbook of Psychooncology*, ed. J. Holland & J. Rowland. New York: Oxford University Press.

Prevost, F. (1976), *Mein Leben beginnt noch einmal.* [*My Life Starts Over Again*]. Freiburg: Herder.

Rank, O. (1914), Der Doppelgaenger, In: *Psychoanalytische Literatur Interpretation*, ed. J. Fischer. Tuebingen: Max Niemeyer, Deutscher Taschenbuch.

_____ (1932), *Art and Artist*. New York: Agathon Press, 1975.

Redd, W. (1989), Management of anticipatory nausea and vomiting. In: *Handbook of Psychooncology*, ed. J. Holland & J. Rowland. New York: Oxford University Press.

Reichstein, R. (1986), *Zimtbaum. Gedichte.* Zuerich: im Waldgut.

_____ (1988), *Lichterloh. Gedichte.* Zurich: im Waltgut.

_____ (1990), Unpublished poem.

Reimann, B. (1984), *Die geliebte, die verfluchte Hoffnung.* [*The Loved, The Cursed Hope*]. Darmstadt: Leichterhand.

Rilke, R. (1966), *Poems 1906-26.* London: Hogarth Press.

Robbins, G. A., McDonald, M. & Pack, C. (1983), Delay in the diagnosis and treatment of physicians with cancer. *Cancer*, 6:624-626.

Rollin, B. (1976), *First You Cry.* New York: Warner.

Romm, S. (1983), The Oral Cancer of Sigmund Freud. *Clin. Plastic Surgery*, 10:709-716.

Rose, G. (1980), *The Power of Form.* New York: International Universities Press.

Rosenthal, T. (1973), *How Could I Not Be Among You?,* New York: Persea.

Sattilaro, A. (1982), *Recalled by Life.* Boston: Houghton Mifflin.

Schein, C. (1981), The death of Ivan Ilych. *N. Y. State J. Med.,* March, 416.

Schur, M. (1972). *Freud: Living and Dying.* New York: International Universities Press.

Schwartz, R. (1984), Aufklahrung ueber die Tumordiagnose und Vorwissen bei Patientinnen unter Bruskrebs verdacht. *Psychother. Med. Psychol.* 34:111-115.

Schwerin, D. (1988), *Diary of a Pigeon Watcher.* New York: Paragon House.

Searles, H. (1981), Psychoanalytic therapy with cancer patients. In: *Psychotherapeutic Treatment of Cancer Patients*, ed. J. Goldberg. New York: Free Press.

Segal, H. (1952), Psychoanalytic approach to aesthetics. *Internat. J. Psycho-Anal.*, 31:196-206.

_____ (1973), *Introduction to the Work of Melanie Klein.* New York: Baric.

Sherman, C., Calman, K., Eckhardt, S., Elsebai, I., Firat,D., Hossfeld,D., Paunier, J., & Salvadori, B., ed. (1987), *Manual of Clinical Oncology.* Berlin, Western Germany: Springer.

Sikes, S. (1984), Beating the boogeyman. A cancer patient's diary, *Bull. Menn. Clin.* 40lS:293-317.

_____ (1988), Falling off the Matterhorn. *Calyx, 2.*

Sloterdijk, P. (1978), *Literatur und Lebenserfahrung.* Muenchen: Carl Hanser.

Solzhenitsyn, A. (1968), *Cancer Ward.* London: Bodley Head.

Sontag, S. (1977), *Illness as Metaphor*. New York: Ferrar, Straus & Giroux.

Spitz, R. (1965), *The First Year of Life*. New York: International Universities Press.

Stoudemire, A. (1983), The onset and adaptation to cancer: Psychodynamics of an ill physician. *Psychiat.*, 46:377-387.

Tallmer, J. (1989), Strokes of pain, comfort and joy. *New York Post*, June 2.

Tolstoy, L. (1882), *Death of Ivan Ilych*. New York: New American Library, 1960.

Twycross, R. (1984a), Analgesics. *Postgrad. Med. J.*, 60:876-880.

_____ (1984b), Control of pain, *J. Royal Coll. Physicians of London*, 18:32-39.

_____ & Ventafridda, V., ed. (1980), *The Continuing Care of Terminal Cancer Patients*. Oxford: Pergamon Press.

Vollmoeller, W. (1982), Amblante Einzelpsychotherapie bei Krebspatienten. *Onkologie*, 5

Wander, M. (1980), *Leben waer eine prima Alternative* [*Life Would Be a Great Alternative*]. Darmstadt: Samlung Luchterhand.

Webster, H. (1980), *Bulletins from a War*. Washington, DC: Word Works.

Weisman, A. (1972), *On Dying and Denying: A Psychiatric Study of Terminality*. New York: Behavioral Publications.

_____ (1979), *Coping with Cancer*. New York: McGraw-Hill.

Winnicott, D.W. (1958), *Through Paediatrics to Psychoanalysis*. London: Tavistock.

_____ (1965), *The Maturational Process and the Facilitating Environment*. New York: International Universities Press.

_____ (1969), Uebergangsobjekte und Uebergangsphenomene.

_____ *Psyche*, 33:660-682.

_____ (1971), *Playing and Reality*. New York: Basic Books.

_____ (1974), Fears of breakdown. *Internat. Rev. Psycho-Anal.*, 1:103-107.

Zorn, F. (1977), *Mars*. Munich: Kindler.

Selected Readings

ENGLISH LANGUAGE

Alsop, S. (1973), *Stay of Execution*. Philadelphia: Lippincott.

Andres, S. & Steiger, B. (1986), *Stella: One Woman's Victory over Cancer*. Tempe, AZ: Synergy Books.

Bayh, M. (1979), *Marvella: A Personal Journey*. New York: Harcourt Brace Jovanovich.

Berte, R. (1987), *To Speak Again: My Victory Over Throat Cancer*. Greenwich, CT.: Devin Adair.

Bishop, B. (1986), *My Triumph Over Cancer*. New Canaan, CT: Keats.

Blumberg, R. (1982), *Headstrong*. New York: Crown.

Boyd, P. (1985), *The Silent Wound*. Reading, MA: Addison-Wesley.

Brody, J. (1978), *You Can Fight Cancer and Win*. New York: McGraw-Hill.

Brooks, S. (1973), *The Cancer Story*. New York: Quality Paperbacks.

Brown, J. (1900), *Terry Fox: A Pictorial Tribute to the Marathon of Hope*. Canada: Paper Jacks.

Buchanan, W. (1979), *A Shining Season*. Albuquerque: University of New Mexico Press.

Cler, A. & Pendelton, B. (1987), *Cancer, God and I and a Natural Cure*. New York: Vantage.

Cook, S. (1982), *Second Life*. New York: Simon & Schuster.

Ford, B. & Chase, C. (1978), *The Times of My Life*. New York: Harper & Row.

Geier, M. (1985), *Cancer: What's It Doing in My Life?* Pasadena, CA: Hope.

Gonte, M. (1987), *It Can't Happen To Me*. Southfield, MI: Marnik.

Graham, J. (1983), *In the Company of Others*. New York: Harcourt Brace Jovanovich.

Helman, E. (1986), *A Life: How a Surgeon Faced His Fatal Illness*. New York: Faber & Faber.

Higginbotham, M. (1974), *With Each Passing Moment*. Tampa, FL: Grace.

Howe, H. (1982), *Do Not Go Gentle*. New York: Norton.

Ireland, J. (1987), *Life Wish*. Boston, MA: Little, Brown,

James, A. (1964), *The Diary of Alice James*, ed. L. Edel. New York: Dodd Mead.

Jones, I. (1986), *I'm Dying and You Don't Know What to Say*. New York: Vantage Press.

Kelli O. (1980), *Until Tomorrow Comes*. Everest House.

Lee, L. (1977), *Walking Through the Fire: A Hospital Journal*. New York: Dutton.

Lorde. A. (1980), *The Cancer Journals*. New York: Spinsters/Aunt Lute.

Lovato, R. (1977), *All the Days of My Life*. Palos Verdes, CA: Morgan Press.

Metzger, D. (1978), *The Woman Who Slept with Men to Take the War Out of Them and Tree*. Berkeley, CA: Wingbow Press.

Michie, M. (1980), "A splendid day," *Virginia Quart. Rev.*, 56:140-423.

Mullan, F. (1983), *Vital Signs*. New York: Farrar, Straus & Giroux.

Murphy, R. (1987), *The Body Silent*. New York: Holt.

Nethery, S. (1978), *One Year and Counting: Breast Cancer, My World and Me*. Grand Rapids, MI: Baker.

Pepper, C. (1984), *We the Victors*. Garden City, NY.: Doubleday.

Pradeau, J. (1976), *I Had This Little Cancer*. New York: Crowell.

Radner, G. (1989), *It's Always Something*. New York: Simon & Schuster.

Rollin, B. (1976), *First You Cry*. New York: New American Library.

Rosenthal. (1973), *How Could I Not Be Among You?* New York: Persea Books.

Rossi, N. (1983), *From This Day Forward*. New York: New York Times.

Ryan, C. & Ryan, K. (1979), *A Private Battle*. New York: Simon & Schuster.

Sanes, S. (1978), *A Physician Faces Cancer Himself*. Albany: New York State University Press.

Sarton, M. (1978), *A Reckoning*. New York: Norton.

_____ (1980), *Recovering*. New York: Norton.

Sattilaro A. (1982), *Recalled by Life*. Boston, MA: Houghton Mifflin.

Schwerin, D. (1988), *Diary of a Pigeon Watcher*. New York: Paragon House.

Seed, P. (1983), *Another Day*. New York: Heinemann.

Sikes, S. (1984), "Beating the boogeyman". A cancer patient's diary, *Bull. Menn. Clin.* 48:293-317.

_____ (1987/88), Falling off the Matterhorn. *Colyx*, 2:80-86.

Simpson, M., Martin, F. (1976), *Coping with Cancer (One Person's Courageous Fight)*. Nashville, TN: Broadman Press.

Smith, M. (1987), *The Shining Eyes of Dawn*. Nopoly Press.

Solkoff, J. (1983), *Learning to Live Again: My Triumph Over Cancer*. New York: Holt.

Solzhenitsyn, A. (1968), *Cancer Ward*. London: Bodley Head.

Spingarn D. (1982), *Hanging in There: Living Well on Borrowed Time*. New York: Stein & Day.

Svenison, K. (1978), *Learning to Live With Cancer*. St Martin's Press.

Troll, P. (1983), *On With My Life*. New York: Putnam.

Tsongas, P. (1984), *Heading Home*. New York: Knopf.

Watson, D. (1985), *Fear No Evil: One Man Deals With Terminal Illness*. Shaw.

Weingarten, V. (1978), *Intimations of Mortality*. New York: Random House.

GERMAN LANGUAGE

Benedict, I. (1987), *Lass mir meine bunten Farben*. West Germany: Bastei Lubbe (Taschenbuch).

Beutler, M. (1980), *Fussfassen*. Bern: Zytglogge.

Cuneo, A. (1982), *Eine Messerspitze Blau*. Zurich: Limmat.

Diggelmann, W.M. (1979), *Schatten Tagebucheine Krankheit*. Zurich: Benziger.

_____ (1980), *Spaziergange auf der Margereteninsel* Erzaehlungen. Zurich: Benziger.

Friebel-Rohring. (1985), *Ich Habe Krebs! Na und?* Rastatt: Hebel.

Hauri D. (1982), *Ich Habe den Herbst gesehen*. Basel: Mond-Buch.

Hosch, T. (1986), *Krebs von Januar bis August?* Stationen einer Morbus-Hodgkin-Erkrankung Heidelberg: Verlag fur Medizin.

Lenker, C. (1984), *Krebs kann auch eine Chance sein*. Frankfurt. Fischer (Taschenbuch).

Noll, P. (1984), *Diktate uber Sterben und Tod*. Munich: Serie Piper.

Pedretti, E. (1986), *Valerie oder das unerzogene Auge*. Frankfurt: Suhrkamp.

Prevost, F. (1976), *Mein Leben beginnt noch einmal*. Freiburg: Herder.

Reimann, B. (1984), *Die geliebte, die verfluchte Hoffnung*. Darmstadt: Luchterhand.

Sandkorn, A. (1986), *Das Signal oder die Entfernung eines Knotens*. Frankfurt: Fischer.

Schnurre, M., Kreibich-Fischer, R. (1987), *Ich will fliegen, leben, tanzen*. Freiburg: Herder Frauenforum.

Van Heyst. L. (1980), *Das schlimmste war die Angst*. Hamburg: Fischer.

Wander, M. (1980), *Leben waer eine prima Alternative*. Sammlung Luchtehand, 1980.

Zorn, F. (1977), *Mars*. Muenchen: Kindler.

SCIENTIFIC CONTRIBUTIONS WRITTEN BY CANCER PATIENTS

Elias, N. (1987), *The Loneliness of the Dying*. Oxford, UK: Basil Blackwell.

Fiore, N. (1987), Fighting cancer—one patient's perspective, *New Eng. J. Med.*, 300:284-289.

_____ (1984), *The Road Back to Health: Coping with the Emotional Side of Cancer*. New York: Bantam.

Kushner, R. (1975), *Breast Cancer: A Personal History and an Investigative Report*. New York: Harcourt Brace Jovanovich.

Pao, P.N. (1983), Suspension of the reality principle in adaptation and in creativity. *Psychoanal. Inq.*, 3:431-449.

Silver, A. (1982), Resuming the work with a life-threatening illness. *Contemp. Psychoanal.* 18:314-326.

Sontag, S. (1977), *Illness as Metaphor*. Farrar, Straus & Giroux.

Stoudemire, A. (1983), The onset and adaptation to cancer: Psychodynamics of an ill physician. *Psychiat.*, 46:377-387.

ENGLISH AND GERMAN POETRY

Badruddin, K. (1982), *Poems of Gitanjali*. London: Oriel Press.

Kovner, A. (1987), *Sloan Kettering, Poems*. Ramat-Gan, Israel: Hakibbutz Hameuchad.

Lifshitz, L. ed. (1988), *Her Soul Beneath the Bone: Women's Poetry on Breast Cancer*, Chicago: University of Illinois Press.

Murray, M. (1974), *The Great Mother and Other Poems*, New York: Sheed & Ward.

Reichstein, R. (1986), *Zimmtbaum. Gedichte*. Wald: Im Waldgut.

_____ (1988), *Lichterloh. Gedichte*. Wald: Im Waldgut.

Sullam, E. (1987), *Out of Bounds*. Potomac, MD: Scripta Humanistica.

Van de Walle, E. (1984), *Falling from Grace*. Vancouver, BC: Press Gang.

Vanessapress, Ed. (1986), *Bits of Ourselves: Woman's Experiences with Cancer*. Fairbanks, AK: Vanessapress.

Webster, H. (1980), *Bulletins from a War*. Washington, DC: Word Works.

Zadravec, K. (1980), *Shewski's Ladder*. Chevy Chase, MD: Primrose Press.

_____ (1986), *How to Travel*. College Park, MD: SCOP Public.

INDEX

DATE DUE